AF885040

Independent CV-BC Exam Study Guide 2027-2028:

600 Updated Practice Questions with Detailed Explanations for the ANCC Cardiac-Vascular Nursing Certification

Caldwell Abiodun

📚 STUDY GUIDE BONUS MATERIAL

🎧 Full Audio Edition

Access the complete book in audio format
Ideal for learning during travel, workouts, or downtime
Stay productive even when you're not in the mood to read

📱 Digital Flashcards

Fast and effective revision tool
Strengthen memory of important concepts
Study anytime, wherever you are

⚡ Quick & Easy Access

No sign-up needed
Compatible with all devices
Smooth and instant usability

📍 ***Access all bonus content on Page 17***

Author Introduction

Cardiac-vascular nursing demands clinical precision, rapid assessment skills, and an in-depth understanding of complex cardiovascular conditions. Certification in Cardiac-Vascular Nursing signifies advanced expertise in caring for patients with acute and chronic cardiac disorders, vascular diseases, and related complications. This study guide has been developed by an experienced cardiovascular nurse in collaboration with a team of critical care specialists, nurse educators, and certification preparation experts dedicated to supporting candidates pursuing specialty recognition in cardiac-vascular nursing.

The lead author brings extensive experience in telemetry, intensive care, cardiac step-down units, and vascular specialty settings. Cardiac-vascular nurses must interpret hemodynamic data, recognize arrhythmias, manage pharmacologic therapies, and respond swiftly to life-threatening changes in patient status. In addition, they provide education, coordinate multidisciplinary care, and support patients and families navigating complex treatment plans. This guide reflects those responsibilities by translating advanced cardiovascular science and clinical practice into structured, exam-focused preparation aligned with the standards established by the American Nurses Credentialing Center (ANCC).

Working collaboratively, the contributing team conducted a comprehensive review of the cardiac-vascular nursing certification content outline to ensure balanced coverage of its major domains. These include cardiovascular anatomy and pathophysiology; acute coronary syndromes; heart failure management; vascular disorders; pharmacologic interventions; invasive and noninvasive diagnostics; and evidence-based practice principles. Each chapter integrates foundational physiology with applied clinical scenarios that reflect real-world patient care challenges.

Recognizing that certification candidates are often practicing nurses balancing demanding clinical responsibilities, this study guide is intentionally structured for clarity and efficiency. Complex hemodynamic concepts, medication protocols, and procedural standards are presented in organized, accessible language without sacrificing clinical depth. Case-based questions, rhythm interpretation exercises, and focused review tools are incorporated to strengthen retention and build exam readiness.

Above all, this resource reflects deep respect for the vital role cardiac-vascular nurses play in improving patient outcomes and advancing cardiovascular care. Achieving specialty certification represents more than passing an examination—it signifies professional excellence, advanced clinical competence, and a steadfast commitment to delivering high-quality, patient-centered care.

Table of Contents

This material is provided for educational and informational purposes only. While every effort has been made to ensure the accuracy, completeness, and reliability of the information presented at the time of publication, the publisher and contributors make no representations or warranties, express or implied, regarding the content. Examination objectives, eligibility requirements, testing formats, regulatory standards, and scoring methodologies may change at the discretion of the relevant certifying or governing organizations. Readers are solely responsible for verifying current information directly with the appropriate official sources before relying on this publication.

This study guide does not constitute legal, medical, financial, or professional advice. It is intended to supplement official resources, structured coursework, and professional training programs—not to replace them. The publisher does not guarantee examination success, certification, licensure, employment, or advancement. Individual results will vary based on preparation, prior knowledge, and testing conditions.

All trademarks, certification marks, service marks, trade names, logos, and registered marks referenced in this publication are the property of their respective owners. Their use is strictly for identification and informational purposes and does not imply endorsement, sponsorship, or affiliation with this publication.

For permissions, licensing, translation rights, or bulk purchase inquiries, please contact the publisher through authorized communication channels.

Disclaimer

CV-BC® is a registered trademark of the American Nurses Credentialing Center. This publication is an independent study tool and is not affiliated with or endorsed by ANCC .

Chapter 1: Assessment and Diagnosis

The practice of cardiac-vascular nursing begins with systematic assessment—collecting, validating, and interpreting data to identify actual and potential problems affecting cardiovascular function. Skilled assessment links pathophysiology with clinical observation, translating physiologic variations into diagnostic reasoning. The nurse's ability to recognize subtle changes often determines how rapidly life-threatening events are averted or mitigated.

Anatomy and Physiology

Understanding the integrated structure of the heart and vasculature is foundational. The cardiac cycle involves a coordinated sequence of electrical and mechanical events: depolarization initiates atrial contraction, followed by ventricular systole, closure of atrioventricular valves, ejection through semilunar valves, and diastolic filling. Coronary perfusion occurs primarily during diastole, emphasizing the vulnerability of tachycardic states to ischemia. Vascular tone, regulated by autonomic input and endothelial mediators such as nitric oxide and endothelin, maintains systemic resistance.

In clinical assessment, nurses correlate these physiologic principles with findings such as jugular venous pressure, pulse contour, and peripheral perfusion. For example, a rapid upstroke and collapsing pulse suggest increased stroke volume and widened pulse pressure as seen in aortic regurgitation, whereas a delayed, diminished pulse indicates outflow obstruction typical of aortic stenosis. Recognizing these tactile and visual cues allows bedside identification of mechanical inefficiencies without immediate reliance on imaging.

Pathophysiology

Cardiovascular disorders arise from structural, electrical, or functional abnormalities that disturb the relationship between oxygen supply and metabolic demand. Atherosclerosis remains the central mechanism for coronary and peripheral artery disease. It evolves from endothelial injury leading to lipid infiltration, inflammatory cell recruitment, and plaque formation. Rupture of unstable plaques precipitates thrombosis, resulting in acute coronary syndromes or cerebrovascular events.

Heart failure exemplifies the continuum from compensatory adaptation to decompensation. According to the 2024 ACC/AHA Performance and Quality Measures, early identification of structural heart disease and neurohormonal activation guides evidence-based interventions. Elevated natriuretic peptide levels, diminished ejection fraction, and imaging evidence of ventricular remodeling inform both staging and prognosis. The nurse synthesizes these findings to prioritize interventions, anticipate complications, and coordinate multidisciplinary input.

Hypertension, redefined under the 2025 AHA/ACC Guideline, remains a leading modifiable determinant of cardiovascular morbidity. Accurate measurement techniques—validated automated devices, appropriate cuff size, and standardized patient positioning—are critical. Out-of-office monitoring (ambulatory or home) confirms diagnosis and distinguishes white-coat or masked hypertension. Nurses play a central role in educating patients about measurement accuracy and adherence to monitoring schedules.

Nursing Diagnosis Identification

Diagnostic reasoning translates assessment data into nursing diagnoses that direct care. Typical examples in cardiac-vascular practice include: decreased cardiac output related to impaired myocardial contractility; excess fluid volume related to compromised regulatory mechanisms; and activity intolerance associated with imbalance between oxygen supply and demand. Each diagnosis integrates objective findings such as abnormal heart sounds, arrhythmias, or edema with subjective symptoms like fatigue or dyspnea.

The diagnostic phase extends beyond labeling; it forms the intellectual bridge between data and planning. Using the ANCC domain model, nurses validate suspected problems through correlation of physiologic evidence, laboratory results, and patient narratives. The outcome is a prioritized list of nursing diagnoses that anticipate acute deterioration while addressing chronic adaptation.

Patient Interview

Comprehensive interviewing elicits both biomedical and psychosocial dimensions. A structured approach begins with the chief complaint—often chest pain, dyspnea, or palpitations—then explores onset, character, precipitating and relieving factors, and associated symptoms. Social determinants such as financial constraints, housing stability, and cultural health beliefs shape adherence and access. Incorporating these factors aligns with contemporary performance measures emphasizing equity in cardiovascular care.

Active listening, empathy, and non-verbal observation reveal cues about anxiety, denial, or health literacy that affect outcomes. Documenting exact medication use, including herbal supplements, is essential to avoid interactions. For instance, concurrent intake of St. John's wort may reduce plasma concentration of certain anticoagulants, heightening thrombotic risk. Through precise interviewing, the nurse establishes rapport and gathers data that later guide diagnostic interpretation and individualized education.

Cardiac-Vascular Assessment Techniques and Tools

Physical assessment integrates inspection, palpation, percussion, and auscultation with advanced monitoring technology. The sequence begins with vital signs—blood pressure in both arms, heart rate, respiratory pattern, temperature, and oxygen saturation. Orthostatic measurements reveal autonomic or volume abnormalities. Inspection of precordium for heaves or pulsations, palpation of apical impulse, and auscultation of heart sounds provide information on chamber size and valvular integrity.

Modern nursing practice extends these fundamentals using Doppler studies to assess peripheral flow, ankle-brachial indices for peripheral arterial disease, and stroke scales to detect neurologic deficits secondary to embolic events. When interpreting cardiac rhythms, recognition of ischemic changes or conduction blocks allows prompt initiation of evidence-based interventions such as rapid reperfusion activation or electrolyte correction.

Data Collection and Interpretation

Comprehensive data collection synthesizes laboratory, imaging, and physiologic information. Serum biomarkers—including troponins, natriuretic peptides, and lipid profiles—guide acute and chronic management. Diagnostic imaging such as echocardiography quantifies ejection fraction, wall motion, and valvular function, while cardiac catheterization delineates anatomic lesions and hemodynamics. According to *Diagnostic Methods in the Cardiac Catheterization Laboratory*, nurses involved in invasive procedures ensure patient safety through pre-procedure verification, continuous monitoring, and recognition of complications like contrast-induced nephropathy or access-site bleeding.

Interpretation requires understanding of normal ranges and clinical context. An elevated troponin in a patient with renal insufficiency demands correlation with ECG and symptoms to differentiate chronic elevation from acute injury. Likewise, abnormal hemodynamic waveforms during catheterization may signify mechanical obstruction or technical artifact. The nurse's analytical capacity ensures that data contribute to meaningful diagnostic conclusions rather than isolated numbers.

Integrating Assessment Findings

Effective diagnosis emerges when findings from diverse sources converge into a coherent picture. A patient presenting with exertional dyspnea, displaced apical impulse, elevated BNP, and echocardiographic evidence of reduced ejection fraction leads logically to the nursing diagnosis of decreased cardiac output secondary to systolic dysfunction. The nurse anticipates related problems—activity intolerance, fluid volume excess, impaired gas exchange—and collaborates on a comprehensive care plan.

Integration also includes recognition of psychosocial patterns. Depression and anxiety frequently accompany cardiovascular illness and adversely affect adherence. Screening tools such as PHQ-9 or GAD-7 provide quantitative assessment that supports holistic diagnosis. Cultural assessment identifies beliefs about illness causation or traditional remedies that may influence medication adherence.

Clinical Example

Consider an adult patient admitted with acute shortness of breath and peripheral edema. Assessment reveals elevated jugular venous pressure, bilateral rales, BNP 1,500 pg/mL, and chest radiograph showing pulmonary congestion. ECG displays sinus tachycardia without ischemic changes. Nursing diagnosis: decreased cardiac output related to impaired myocardial contractility secondary to chronic heart failure. Interventions initially focus on positioning to enhance ventilation, administering prescribed diuretics, monitoring urine output, and evaluating weight trends. Simultaneously, the nurse provides emotional reassurance and explains the relationship between fluid retention and symptoms, preparing the patient for subsequent self-management education.

Correlation of Diagnostic Findings

After data are collected, correlation ensures that physiological, biochemical, and behavioral evidence align to support or refute possible diagnoses. Correlation converts fragments of data into a clinically meaningful pattern. When nurses interpret a patient's weight gain, elevated jugular venous pressure, and rising BNP together, they confirm fluid overload rather than treating each finding in isolation.

Correlation also detects contradictions—such as an echocardiogram indicating preserved ejection fraction while the patient exhibits profound fatigue and orthopnea—prompting exploration of diastolic dysfunction or pulmonary pathology.

Risk stratification integrates these correlations into predictive models that identify patients at high likelihood of deterioration. Contemporary performance measures from the American Heart Association emphasize early risk identification using scores such as TIMI, GRACE, or CHA_2DS_2-VASc. Although these tools were developed for medical use, nurses apply their logic in triage and care coordination. Recognizing that a patient with elevated troponin, hypotension, and renal impairment falls into a higher risk category guides the urgency of intervention and interprofessional communication.

Interpretation of Rhythm and Hemodynamic Data

Continuous ECG monitoring remains a cornerstone of cardiac-vascular nursing. Nurses identify patterns that predict instability—progressive prolongation of PR intervals, premature ventricular contractions in runs, or conversion from sinus rhythm to atrial fibrillation. Understanding the physiologic meaning behind these changes allows timely initiation of guideline-directed interventions. For example, detection of new-onset atrial fibrillation in a hypertensive patient initiates anticoagulation evaluation and rate control per current practice recommendations.

Invasive and non-invasive hemodynamic data provide deeper insight into circulatory performance. When interpreting pulmonary artery pressures or cardiac output measurements, nurses correlate numeric values with clinical presentation. A reduced cardiac index in the presence of low systemic vascular resistance indicates distributive shock, whereas the same index with elevated filling pressures suggests cardiogenic failure. Recognizing these nuances prevents inappropriate fluid administration or vasodilator therapy.

Cultural and Ethical Dimensions of Diagnosis

Assessment extends beyond biophysical data to include cultural meaning and ethical context. Many patients interpret cardiac disease through spiritual or familial frameworks. A thorough diagnostic process respects these perspectives while ensuring that care remains evidence-based. Ethical sensitivity is essential when disclosing prognostic information or obtaining consent for invasive diagnostics. Nurses balance respect for autonomy with beneficence, explaining procedures in language appropriate to literacy level and cultural background.

Hemodynamic Physiology in Clinical Context

Precise interpretation of hemodynamic data distinguishes expert cardiac-vascular nurses. Every pressure tracing conveys a physiologic story. The a-wave on a right-atrial tracing reflects atrial contraction; an absent a-wave in atrial fibrillation illustrates mechanical-electrical dissociation. Elevated v-waves suggest tricuspid regurgitation, while a steep y-descent signals restrictive filling. When the nurse correlates waveform morphology with clinical findings—jugular distention, hepatomegaly, and peripheral edema—the diagnostic picture becomes three-dimensional.

Left-sided pressures complete the hemodynamic narrative. An increased pulmonary-capillary wedge pressure accompanied by normal cardiac output indicates isolated diastolic dysfunction; when coupled with diminished output, it defines systolic failure. Through trend analysis rather than isolated numbers, nurses anticipate escalation toward pulmonary congestion or low-output shock and mobilize interventions before critical thresholds are reached.

Advanced Electrocardiographic Interpretation

Beyond rhythm recognition, advanced ECG analysis detects conduction abnormalities, ischemic injury, and electrolyte disturbances. ST-segment elevation in contiguous leads identifies acute transmural ischemia; depression or T-wave inversion signifies subendocardial strain. Prolonged QT intervals demand scrutiny for drug-induced effects or electrolyte imbalance. Nurses versed in these subtleties expedite reperfusion activation and pharmacologic correction, directly influencing survival.

Continuous telemetry generates data streams requiring vigilant pattern appraisal. Trend review—progressive QRS widening in a patient on antiarrhythmic therapy—alerts nurses to potential proarrhythmia. Integration of ECG findings with symptoms such as palpitations, dizziness, or syncope distinguishes benign variants from emergent instability.

Diagnostic Imaging Integration

Modern cardiac-vascular nursing incorporates interpretation of non-invasive imaging reports. Echocardiography remains the cornerstone, offering visualization of chamber size, wall motion, and valvular performance. Understanding ejection fraction thresholds enables nurses to contextualize guideline-directed therapy initiation. For instance, an ejection fraction below forty percent triggers specific pharmacologic pathways, whereas preserved function shifts focus toward diastolic management.

Computed-tomographic angiography and magnetic-resonance imaging extend assessment to structural and perfusion anomalies. Nurses ensure appropriate preparation—hydration for contrast protection, removal of metal objects for MRI safety—and translate results into patient language. "The scan shows your heart muscle pumps about half the blood out each beat; we'll work on strengthening that efficiency through medication and activity."

Biomarker Evolution and Interpretation

Biochemical markers continually evolve as diagnostic tools. High-sensitivity troponin assays detect minute myocardial injury earlier than previous generations. Understanding kinetics—rise within hours, plateau, and gradual decline—prevents misinterpretation of chronically elevated values in renal impairment. Nurses coordinate serial draws and communicate trends, recognizing that pattern, not a single value, confirms diagnosis.

Inflammatory and metabolic markers, including C-reactive protein and lipoprotein(a), refine risk profiling. Nurses educate patients on lifestyle implications, explaining how weight control, smoking cessation, and lipid management influence these indices. Bridging laboratory science with behavior change exemplifies the nurse's translational role.

Integrating Genomic and Precision-Medicine Data

Emerging precision-medicine approaches identify genetic polymorphisms affecting drug metabolism and disease susceptibility. Testing for CYP2C19 variants informs antiplatelet therapy selection after percutaneous intervention. Nurses ensure informed consent, clarify the scope of testing, and integrate results into documentation. As genomic data enter practice, ethical stewardship—protecting privacy and preventing discrimination—becomes part of diagnostic professionalism.

Multisystem Correlation

Cardiac disease rarely exists in isolation. Renal, pulmonary, and endocrine interactions shape diagnostic complexity. In heart-failure patients, rising creatinine may signal renal congestion rather than intrinsic nephropathy; recognizing this prevents premature discontinuation of life-saving medications. Pulmonary findings—wheezes versus crackles—differentiate bronchospasm from volume overload. Thyroid dysfunction alters rhythm and contractility; routine screening identifies reversible causes of arrhythmia or heart failure.

Through integrated assessment, nurses create holistic diagnoses that acknowledge interdependence among organ systems.

Diagnostic Decision-Making Under Uncertainty

Real-world assessment often involves ambiguity: inconclusive tests, overlapping symptoms, or limited data. Expert nurses navigate uncertainty through probabilistic reasoning—assigning likelihood rather than seeking absolutes. They weigh pre-test probability, test sensitivity, and specificity to judge reliability. For example, a negative stress test in a patient with high pre-test probability of coronary disease warrants further imaging rather than reassurance.

Clinical intuition complements analytic reasoning. Subtle cues—restlessness, pallor, sweating—may precede measurable deterioration. Trusting experiential knowledge while verifying objectively epitomizes advanced diagnostic artistry.

Cultural and Psychosocial Determinants of Diagnostic Accuracy

Cultural perception influences symptom reporting. Some populations describe chest pain as "pressure" or "indigestion," delaying recognition. Gender differences further complicate interpretation; women often present with atypical manifestations. Nurses counter these disparities by probing beyond surface descriptions, using open questions and culturally appropriate metaphors.

Psychosocial factors, including health beliefs and stigma, affect disclosure. A patient minimizing dyspnea to avoid burdening family may withhold critical information. Establishing trust through empathy enhances diagnostic completeness.

Safety in Diagnostic Procedures

Every diagnostic step entails risk. Contrast nephropathy, radiation exposure, and vascular complications demand prevention strategies. Pre-procedure screening for allergies, renal function, and pregnancy ensures safety. During procedures, nurses monitor vital signs, consciousness level, and comfort, intervening promptly for hypotension or arrhythmia. Post-procedure care includes hydration, site inspection, and patient education on warning signs of complication.

Safety extends to infection prevention during invasive monitoring. Strict adherence to sterile technique and device maintenance minimizes catheter-related bloodstream infections. Documentation of compliance aligns with institutional quality measures.

Case Study: Complex Diagnostic Synthesis

A middle-aged patient presents with episodic chest tightness and exertional fatigue. Resting ECG normal; troponin slightly elevated; echocardiogram reveals mild diastolic dysfunction. Nurse correlates findings, noting uncontrolled hypertension and anemia. Recognizing multifactorial etiology—supply-demand mismatch rather than plaque rupture—she advocates for blood-pressure optimization and anemia correction. Subsequent improvement without ischemic evidence confirms diagnostic accuracy derived from comprehensive assessment.

Reflection and Professional Growth

Diagnostic mastery evolves through reflection. After each case, nurses review outcomes against initial impressions, identifying cognitive biases—anchoring on first impressions or overreliance on technology. Journaling and peer discussion transform experience into expertise. Participation in morbidity-mortality reviews enhances collective learning, embedding safety culture.

Integration With Educational and Leadership Roles

Advanced diagnostic skill positions nurses as educators for peers and students. Demonstrating correlation of findings, guiding new staff through rhythm analysis, and explaining hemodynamic reasoning elevate unit competence. Leadership in assessment rounds fosters standardization and early recognition of deterioration.

Technology and Artificial-Intelligence Support

Machine-learning algorithms now assist with ECG interpretation and imaging analysis. Nurses remain critical gatekeepers, validating algorithmic suggestions against clinical context. Understanding model limitations—training bias, false positives—prevents blind reliance. Collaboration with informatics teams ensures that digital tools augment rather than replace professional judgment.

Ethical Considerations in Data Use

The expansion of digital diagnostics introduces privacy and consent challenges. Nurses safeguard patient data, ensuring that remote-monitoring transmissions occur through encrypted channels. Transparent explanation of data use builds trust. When results reveal incidental findings, nurses guide disclosure in consultation with the care team, balancing beneficence with respect for autonomy.

Access Audio file and Flashcards

Scan QR Code Below

Chapter 2: Planning and Implementation

Planning translates diagnostic insight into coordinated actions that restore or maintain cardiovascular stability. Implementation then transforms those plans into real-time interventions. This domain, representing thirty-five percent of the examination content, evaluates a nurse's ability to integrate guidelines, ethics, and multidisciplinary collaboration into direct patient care.

Evidence-Based Practice Guidelines

Current practice relies on evidence synthesized by professional societies such as the ACC and AHA. The 2024 update of the Heart Failure Performance and Quality Measures and the 2025 Hypertension Guideline provide the backbone for modern cardiovascular planning. Nurses must internalize the rationale behind these recommendations rather than memorize numeric targets. For instance, the emphasis on achieving blood-pressure goals through combined lifestyle and pharmacologic strategies reflects data linking even modest reductions in systolic pressure to significant decreases in stroke and myocardial infarction risk.

When constructing care plans, the nurse aligns patient-specific goals with these national standards. A plan for a patient with heart failure with reduced ejection fraction includes optimization of guideline-directed medical therapy—angiotensin receptor-neprilysin inhibitors, beta-blockers, mineralocorticoid receptor antagonists, and SGLT2 inhibitors—while concurrently addressing diet, fluid balance, and physical conditioning. Nurses monitor for side effects, reinforce adherence, and advocate for medication titration consistent with evidence thresholds.

Scope and Standards of Practice

Cardiac-vascular nursing operates within defined professional boundaries established by national scope and standards statements. Planning begins with recognition of what nursing independently manages and where collaboration or referral is required. For example, adjusting oxygen delivery systems or initiating patient education lies squarely within nursing practice, while modification of invasive device settings requires physician authorization. Maintaining this distinction preserves patient safety and professional accountability.

Interprofessional collaboration is embedded in planning. Effective communication with physicians, pharmacists, dietitians, and physical therapists ensures that the plan addresses all determinants of cardiovascular health. Structured tools such as SBAR (Situation-Background-Assessment-Recommendation) standardize handoffs and reduce error. Nurses take leadership in coordinating multidisciplinary rounds, presenting concise yet complete data that drive collective decision-making.

Legal and Ethical Considerations

Ethical and legal vigilance permeate every phase of planning and implementation. Informed consent demands that patients receive understandable information regarding risks, benefits, and alternatives to procedures or medications. Documentation must verify comprehension rather than mere signature collection. Confidentiality remains paramount when discussing cardiovascular risk factors such as lifestyle or genetic predispositions.

Advance directives guide care when patients lose decision-making capacity. Nurses initiate these discussions early, framing them as proactive planning rather than crisis management. Ethical dilemmas often arise when patient preferences conflict with clinical recommendations—for example, refusal of anticoagulation due to fear of bleeding. The nurse's role is to explore underlying concerns, provide balanced information, and support autonomous choice while ensuring that refusal is informed.

Invasive and Non-Invasive Procedures

Planning for procedures requires detailed pre-, intra-, and post-care coordination. Non-invasive diagnostics such as echocardiography, nuclear imaging, or computed tomography require patient preparation to optimize image quality—fasting, medication adjustment, and explanation of sensations expected during the test. Invasive interventions, including cardiac catheterization or electrophysiologic studies, demand sterile preparation, allergy assessment for contrast media, and verification of renal function.

According to *Diagnostic Methods in the Cardiac Catheterization Laboratory*, the nurse ensures that informed consent is obtained, monitors vital signs and ECG continuously, and recognizes early signs of complications such as arrhythmias, hypotension, or access-site bleeding. Post-procedure, assessment focuses on hemostasis, distal perfusion, and return of consciousness. Prompt recognition of retroperitoneal hemorrhage or contrast reaction exemplifies critical nursing vigilance.

Surgical Interventions

Planning extends to perioperative and postoperative care of patients undergoing cardiac or vascular surgery. For coronary artery bypass grafting, valve replacement, or transplantation, preoperative teaching reduces anxiety and improves postoperative outcomes. Key elements include explanation of incision care, pulmonary hygiene, and activity progression. During immediate postoperative care, nurses manage hemodynamic monitoring lines, maintain normothermia, and titrate vasoactive medications in coordination with the critical-care team.

Knowledge of expected recovery trajectories distinguishes normal adaptation from complication. For instance, transient low-grade fever following cardiopulmonary bypass may reflect inflammatory response rather than infection, while sudden output changes from chest tubes demand immediate evaluation for tamponade. Integrating such detail into care plans demonstrates advanced clinical reasoning expected of certified cardiac-vascular nurses.

Pharmacologic Therapies

Implementation of pharmacologic therapy constitutes a substantial component of this domain. Understanding mechanisms of action, therapeutic goals, and adverse reactions allows nurses to administer and evaluate medications safely. Antihypertensives, antiarrhythmics, anticoagulants, and lipid-lowering agents each require specific monitoring parameters.

The 2025 Hypertension Guideline emphasizes individualized targets and combination therapy for resistant hypertension. Nurses educate patients about dosing schedules, side-effect recognition, and the importance of consistent follow-up. Monitoring for orthostatic hypotension, electrolyte imbalance, or renal dysfunction prevents adverse events. Similarly, in heart failure management, adherence to beta-blocker titration schedules is essential; abrupt withdrawal can precipitate decompensation.

Polypharmacy introduces complex interactions. Concurrent administration of ACE inhibitors and potassium-sparing diuretics necessitates vigilance for hyperkalemia. The nurse reconciles all medications, verifies laboratory results, and communicates potential conflicts to the prescriber. Continuous patient teaching reinforces understanding of purpose and expected outcomes, transforming compliance into informed partnership.

Non-Pharmacologic and Complementary Therapies

Lifestyle modification remains foundational to cardiovascular health. Diet planning incorporates sodium restriction, weight management, and lipid control following evidence-based dietary patterns. Exercise prescriptions draw upon cardiac rehabilitation principles—gradual increase in aerobic activity under monitored conditions, progressing to independent maintenance once tolerance improves.

Complementary approaches such as mindfulness, relaxation breathing, and structured stress-management programs have documented benefits in reducing sympathetic activation and blood-pressure variability. Nurses evaluate these practices for safety, avoiding unregulated supplements or energy therapies that may interfere with medical treatment. Integrating validated complementary methods demonstrates holistic care consistent with ANCC standards.

Risk-Reduction Measures

Preventive strategies intersect with every care plan. Venous thromboembolism prophylaxis, infection control, and pressure-injury prevention are universal considerations. For vascular patients, prophylactic anticoagulation or mechanical compression devices minimize clot formation during immobilization. Infection prevention encompasses meticulous catheter-site care and adherence to sterile technique during line insertion or dressing changes.

Education forms a central component of risk reduction. Patients and families learn early warning signs of complications—bleeding, infection, or chest pain—and appropriate responses. Empowering them to recognize and report deviations from expected recovery prevents escalation. Nurses document these teachings as evidence of both quality care and regulatory compliance.

Prioritization and Care Coordination

Effective planning requires triage among competing needs. Nurses apply clinical reasoning frameworks such as Maslow's hierarchy and the ABCs (Airway, Breathing, Circulation) to determine immediate priorities, while long-term planning addresses chronic adaptation. Coordination across transitions of care—hospital to home, acute to rehabilitation—ensures continuity and prevents readmission.

Case management and telehealth technology expand the nurse's ability to monitor patients remotely. Electronic alerts for weight gain or blood-pressure deviation enable early intervention. Communication of findings to the interdisciplinary team closes the feedback loop between patient monitoring and treatment adjustment.

Advanced Cardiovascular Interventions

Planning for advanced interventions requires detailed anticipation of physiologic changes and vigilant post-procedure observation. Implantable cardioverter-defibrillators, pacemakers, and left-ventricular assist devices are increasingly common in cardiac-vascular units. The nurse coordinates multidisciplinary care—cardiology, electrophysiology, and rehabilitation—to ensure safe activation and patient adaptation. Post-implant, nurses monitor device function through telemetry, assess incision sites, and educate patients about magnetic field exposure and remote monitoring.

For patients undergoing percutaneous coronary intervention, nursing implementation centers on maintaining arterial access integrity, observing for reperfusion arrhythmias, and enforcing strict medication adherence. Antiplatelet therapy—dual agents following stent placement—demands consistent education on timing, bleeding precautions, and the consequences of premature discontinuation. Documentation of patient comprehension and adherence tracking demonstrates accountability under performance metrics.

Vascular surgery planning follows similar principles. For carotid endarterectomy, limb bypass, or aneurysm repair, preoperative nursing roles include optimization of blood pressure, glycemic control, and infection prophylaxis. Implementation of postoperative surveillance—neurologic checks, distal pulse monitoring, and wound assessment—enables early recognition of complications such as stroke or graft occlusion.

Hemodynamic and Fluid Management

Effective implementation requires mastery of volume assessment and manipulation. Nurses analyze daily weight, intake and output, hemodynamic pressures, and physical signs such as jugular distention or crackles. Fluid balance plans balance perfusion with congestion risk. In heart failure management, diuretic titration relies on serial weight trends and renal function monitoring.

Electrolyte management integrates with fluid therapy. Hypokalemia from aggressive diuresis can precipitate arrhythmias, whereas hyperkalemia from renal dysfunction or medication interactions threatens conduction stability. Nurses coordinate laboratory testing schedules and communicate critical values promptly. Patient teaching about dietary potassium sources consolidates prevention.

Quality and Safety Initiatives

Implementation is inseparable from quality assurance. National initiatives such as Get With The Guidelines and Magnet Recognition emphasize nursing leadership in improving outcomes. Nurses apply Plan-Do-Study-Act cycles to reduce readmissions, enhance medication reconciliation, or improve blood-pressure control rates. Incorporating these processes into routine care transforms guidelines into measurable performance.

Safety bundles guide specific interventions—central-line insertion, Foley catheter care, and pressure-injury prevention. Nurses verify checklist completion, audit compliance, and analyze near-miss data to sustain continuous improvement. Integration of these measures within everyday workflow reflects the professional maturity expected of board-certified nurses.

Cardiac Rehabilitation Integration

Implementation extends beyond acute treatment to long-term recovery. The *Cardiac Rehabilitation Manual* emphasizes the multidimensional structure of rehabilitation: exercise, nutrition, psychosocial support, and risk-factor modification. Nurses collaborate with physiologists to tailor exercise prescriptions according to functional capacity. Incremental workload increases are guided by heart-rate targets and perceived-exertion scales.

Education on heart-healthy nutrition focuses on reducing saturated fat, controlling sodium, and increasing fiber. Behavioral change techniques—goal setting, self-monitoring, and reinforcement—are interwoven throughout sessions. Nurses monitor vital signs during training, respond to abnormal responses, and document progress. Integration of these components ensures sustainable secondary prevention.

Psychosocial and Behavioral Implementation

Cardiac disease disrupts identity and lifestyle. Planning that ignores psychosocial adjustment risks poor adherence and recurrent events. Nurses implement screening for depression, anxiety, and social isolation, connecting patients with counseling or support groups. Cognitive-behavioral strategies help patients reframe limitations into achievable goals.

Family inclusion strengthens adherence. Teaching sessions that involve spouses or caregivers improve medication management and dietary compliance. Culturally sensitive communication acknowledges traditional healing beliefs while maintaining clinical accuracy. Documentation of family involvement demonstrates holistic implementation in line with professional standards.

Patient Teaching and Literacy Considerations

Effective education is the heart of implementation. Teaching strategies vary according to literacy, language, and learning style. Nurses use plain language, visual aids, and teach-back methods to confirm understanding. For complex regimens such as heart-failure self-management, stepwise instruction—daily weights, symptom logs, when to call for help—anchors behavioral memory.

Technology enhances reach: mobile reminders for medication timing, digital blood-pressure logs, and telehealth coaching extend education beyond discharge. However, privacy and data-security protocols must be observed. Balancing accessibility with confidentiality underscores the ethical dimension of modern nursing practice.

Documentation and Evaluation Within Implementation

Documentation is both legal record and clinical communication tool. Accurate charting of assessments, interventions, and responses ensures continuity. Electronic health records enable trend analysis; structured templates reduce omission. Nurses verify that documentation reflects individualized care rather than generic checklists. Regular review of documentation patterns supports compliance with accreditation standards.

With the implementation phase complete, the nurse transitions naturally into evaluation—measuring whether planned interventions achieved expected outcomes and modifying plans accordingly.

Integrating Evidence-Based Care Pathways

Advanced cardiac-vascular nursing requires translating guideline statements into individualized pathways of care. Evidence-based algorithms for acute coronary syndrome, heart failure, and hypertension provide the structure, but real-world implementation demands adaptation to comorbidities, age, and social context. Certified nurses interpret guideline hierarchies—class of recommendation and level of evidence—to determine intervention priority.

In practice, this may involve aligning acute interventions with chronic goals. A patient admitted for decompensated heart failure benefits from early initiation of long-term therapies while acute symptoms resolve. The nurse ensures that inotropic support transitions smoothly to oral agents as stability returns, coordinating pharmacy education and follow-up scheduling. Evidence becomes actionable through deliberate sequencing of steps that respect both physiology and human factors.

Multidisciplinary Care Coordination

Complex cardiovascular care requires orchestration among multiple disciplines. The nurse assumes a central coordinating role, ensuring that cardiology, endocrinology, nephrology, and rehabilitation efforts remain aligned. Structured interdisciplinary rounds create a shared mental model, reducing duplication and error. The nurse synthesizes information from each specialist into a coherent plan that patients and families can understand.

Effective coordination extends beyond the hospital. Communication with primary-care providers, home-health nurses, and pharmacists ensures continuity. The transition summary prepared by the cardiac-vascular nurse highlights current medications, pending diagnostics, and recommended follow-up intervals. High-quality coordination directly correlates with reduced readmissions and improved patient satisfaction.

Advanced Pharmacologic Management

Pharmacologic planning encompasses selection, titration, and monitoring of complex regimens. Nurses understand the pharmacodynamics and pharmacokinetics underpinning therapy, enabling precise observation for efficacy and toxicity. For instance, when initiating angiotensin receptor–neprilysin inhibitors, the nurse verifies washout of prior ACE inhibitor therapy to prevent angioedema, monitors blood pressure for hypotension, and evaluates renal function within the first week.

In arrhythmia management, antiarrhythmic drugs require meticulous surveillance for QT prolongation and bradycardia. The nurse ensures electrolyte stability and coordinates serial ECGs. Anticoagulant management integrates laboratory and point-of-care testing; education on dietary consistency and interaction avoidance supports safe implementation.

Polypharmacy challenges demand medication reconciliation at every transition. Nurses review herbal and over-the-counter supplements to detect hidden interactions. Clear documentation of medication purpose fosters understanding among all caregivers.

Device and Technology Integration

Planning includes safe use of implantable and external devices. For pacemakers and defibrillators, nurses verify manufacturer specifications, program settings, and patient restrictions regarding electromagnetic interference. Device interrogation data are interpreted collaboratively with electrophysiology teams. Education on remote monitoring empowers patients to participate in surveillance.

Mechanical circulatory support devices such as ventricular assist systems or intra-aortic balloon pumps require advanced technical competence. Nurses monitor hemodynamics, maintain sterility of driveline exits, and adjust anticoagulation protocols. Simulation-based training strengthens team readiness for device emergencies, including power failure or system alarms.

Fluid and Hemodynamic Optimization

Implementation at this level involves dynamic management of preload, afterload, and contractility. Using invasive and noninvasive monitoring, nurses titrate fluids, vasodilators, and inotropes to achieve optimal perfusion. They interpret mixed venous oxygen saturation and cardiac output trends to balance oxygen delivery and demand. Continuous reassessment distinguishes responsive versus refractory states, guiding escalation or de-escalation.

In heart failure, the goal shifts from transient improvement to long-term stability. Nurses educate patients on daily weights, sodium limits, and diuretic timing to sustain fluid equilibrium outside the hospital. The bridge between intensive monitoring and self-management exemplifies holistic implementation.

Behavioral and Psychosocial Integration

Cardiac outcomes hinge on psychosocial adaptation. Nurses embed behavioral assessment into care planning, using validated tools for depression and anxiety. They implement evidence-based interventions—brief cognitive-behavioral counseling, relaxation training, and peer-support referral—to mitigate emotional triggers that compromise adherence.

Motivational interviewing continues throughout hospitalization. By exploring ambivalence and reinforcing self-efficacy, nurses transform prescriptive education into collaborative planning. This interpersonal precision enhances the likelihood that patients will sustain behavior change.

Crisis and Emergency Implementation

Cardiac emergencies test the nurse's capacity for rapid coordination. During cardiac arrest or acute decompensation, nurses apply Advanced Cardiovascular Life Support algorithms with precision, ensuring defibrillation, medication administration, and airway management occur seamlessly. Post-resuscitation care involves targeted temperature management and neurologic assessment.

Leadership during crisis extends beyond task execution to maintaining composure and communication clarity. The nurse leader assigns roles, verbalizes observations, and documents interventions in real time. Post-event debriefing transforms acute stress into learning, fortifying future readiness.

Ethical Decision-Making in Implementation

Ethical challenges emerge when implementing invasive or life-sustaining treatments. Nurses advocate for decisions consistent with patient values and informed consent. When prognosis is poor, discussions about palliative options require honesty tempered with compassion. Maintaining respect for autonomy, even when choices diverge from clinical recommendation, honors professional integrity.

Allocation of limited resources—intensive-care beds, transplant organs—demands transparency and fairness. Nurses contribute to ethical committees, offering the bedside perspective that grounds policy in patient reality. Documentation of ethical deliberation demonstrates accountability and moral courage.

Professional Leadership and Mentorship

Implementation evolves into leadership as nurses mentor colleagues in complex care. They conduct skill workshops on advanced monitoring, interpretive reasoning, and guideline application. Leadership includes evaluating practice gaps and designing training to address them. Coaching new nurses through the emotional demands of high-acuity care sustains workforce resilience.

Mentorship also ensures succession. Experienced nurses model advocacy, professionalism, and reflective practice. By cultivating future leaders, they extend influence beyond individual patients to the profession's growth.

Quality-Improvement Implementation Projects

Certified nurses often spearhead projects translating evidence into practice. Examples include implementing standardized heart-failure discharge checklists or developing electronic alerts for medication contraindications. Nurses gather baseline data, design interventions, and evaluate outcomes through statistical analysis. Results feed back into policy revision, closing the quality loop.

The success of such projects depends on engagement. Nurses employ change-management strategies—communicating rationale, addressing resistance, and celebrating progress. Measurable improvements in metrics validate the initiative and demonstrate the tangible impact of advanced practice.

Integrative and Complementary Therapies

Implementation incorporates validated complementary modalities that enhance recovery and well-being. Structured relaxation, mindfulness meditation, and yoga improve autonomic balance and blood-pressure variability. Nurses evaluate each method's evidence base, ensuring alignment with safety standards and patient preference. Integrating these approaches within conventional regimens exemplifies holistic planning.

Sustainability and Resource Stewardship

Resource stewardship forms part of ethical implementation. Nurses advocate for cost-effective choices that maintain quality: selecting evidence-supported treatments, reducing waste, and optimizing supply use. Awareness of financial implications helps tailor plans to patient affordability, minimizing nonadherence due to cost.

Sustainability also refers to environmental responsibility—proper disposal of medical waste, minimizing single-use plastics when safe alternatives exist, and energy conservation in unit operations. Professional accountability extends to ecological health, recognizing the link between environmental and human cardiovascular well-being.

Chapter 3: Evaluation and Modification

Evaluation determines effectiveness and guides refinement of care. It represents eighteen percent of the examination content and tests the nurse's analytical ability to compare outcomes with expectations, identify variances, and implement corrective strategies.

Outcome Measurement

Outcome evaluation uses objective and subjective criteria. Physiologic indicators—blood-pressure control, lipid levels, weight stability, ejection fraction—quantify physiologic progress. Functional outcomes such as exercise tolerance or return to work assess rehabilitation success. Patient-reported outcomes capture satisfaction, quality of life, and self-efficacy.

Benchmarking aligns individual performance with institutional or national standards. Comparing a unit's rate of post-myocardial-infarction beta-blocker use with national averages reveals areas for quality improvement. Nurses contribute to these databases through accurate data collection and verification.

Continuous Monitoring and Trend Recognition

Ongoing surveillance allows early identification of deviation. Subtle trends—gradual rise in resting heart rate, increased edema, or declining exercise tolerance—may precede acute decompensation. Nurses translate these observations into timely adjustments: modifying diuretic schedules, reinforcing sodium restriction, or escalating evaluation to the provider.

Remote monitoring extends evaluation beyond the hospital. Patients transmit daily weights and blood-pressure readings; nurses analyze data for early warning signs. Prompt telephonic or electronic follow-up reduces readmissions and enhances patient confidence.

Clinical Judgment in Modification

Modification requires synthesis of evidence, experience, and patient preference. When outcomes fail to meet targets, nurses reassess contributing factors—medication adherence, comorbidities, or social barriers. Adjustments might include altering activity levels, re-educating on diet, or coordinating medication review.

Critical thinking distinguishes modification from routine repetition. The nurse examines whether interventions were implemented as planned, whether underlying assumptions remain valid, and whether new evidence necessitates change. This reflective practice embodies professional accountability.

Interdisciplinary Evaluation

Collaborative evaluation strengthens accuracy. During multidisciplinary rounds, nurses present outcome data, patient feedback, and their clinical impressions. Physicians contribute diagnostic interpretation; therapists report functional progress; dietitians analyze nutritional adherence. Joint discussion yields comprehensive modification strategies that address physical, psychological, and environmental dimensions.

Quality-Measure Integration

Modern cardiovascular care ties evaluation directly to performance metrics. The 2024 Heart Failure Performance Measures specify benchmarks for documentation of ejection fraction, prescription of evidence-based medications, and post-discharge follow-up. Nurses track compliance within their units, identify barriers, and participate in corrective action plans. These activities transform individual evaluation into organizational improvement.

Patient Engagement in Evaluation

Evaluation succeeds only when patients share ownership. Teach-back sessions confirm that education produced comprehension. Motivational interviewing explores readiness for lifestyle change and reinforces intrinsic motivation. When patients articulate goals in their own words, outcomes become personally meaningful, sustaining adherence.

Involving patients in self-evaluation—maintaining symptom diaries, logging exercise minutes, and graphing blood-pressure trends—turns monitoring into empowerment. Nurses review these records collaboratively, acknowledging progress and problem-solving setbacks.

Case Illustration

A patient completing six weeks of cardiac rehabilitation demonstrates a ten-percent increase in exercise capacity but reports persistent fatigue. Evaluation reveals suboptimal beta-blocker dosing and inadequate sleep hygiene. The nurse collaborates with the physician to adjust medication, reinforces bedtime routine, and schedules follow-up. At subsequent review, fatigue resolves and exercise endurance improves. This example illustrates cyclical evaluation leading to modification.

Ethical and Legal Dimensions of Evaluation

Accurate reporting of outcomes demands honesty and transparency. Nurses avoid data manipulation for performance appearance; authenticity upholds ethical integrity. When evaluation exposes practice gaps, the professional response is system improvement rather than blame. Documentation of adverse events follows institutional policy to ensure learning and accountability.

Confidentiality persists during evaluation. When presenting cases at quality meetings, identifiers are removed. Respect for patient privacy coexists with the obligation to improve population outcomes.

Documentation of Evaluation and Modification

Clear documentation closes the loop of the nursing process. Entries specify which outcomes were met, partially met, or unmet; what changes were made; and the rationale for modification. Time-stamped progress notes and interdisciplinary summaries create an auditable trail demonstrating professional reasoning.

Continuous learning arises from this process. Each evaluation cycle refines clinical judgment, enhances efficiency, and promotes better outcomes.

Data Analytics and Outcome Interpretation

In advanced practice settings, outcome evaluation increasingly depends on digital data analytics. Electronic health-record dashboards aggregate variables such as medication adherence, readmission rates, and patient-reported quality-of-life scores. The nurse interprets these metrics not as abstract statistics but as reflections of day-to-day care. A sudden spike in readmissions for heart-failure patients may reveal gaps in discharge education or follow-up scheduling. Translating numbers into actions exemplifies analytic competence.

Predictive modeling supports proactive modification. Algorithms incorporating vital-sign trends, laboratory results, and demographic risk factors identify patients at high probability of deterioration. The nurse uses these alerts to initiate preventive interventions—reinforcing sodium restriction, scheduling urgent labs, or arranging early clinic review. The essence of evaluation lies in anticipating change before crisis ensues.

Incorporating Evidence Updates

Continuous modification demands awareness of evolving evidence. When updated guidelines introduce new therapeutic thresholds—such as the expanded role of SGLT2 inhibitors in heart failure or refined blood-pressure targets—nurses reassess current plans. They compare institutional protocols with guideline revisions and advocate for policy alignment. Lifelong learning, journal review, and participation in professional societies maintain currency of practice.

Reflective evaluation also encompasses ethical self-assessment. Nurses examine whether personal bias or cognitive shortcuts influenced earlier planning. Recognizing these patterns promotes humility and intellectual growth.

Transition-of-Care Evaluation

One of the most sensitive phases of cardiovascular care is transition from hospital to home or rehabilitation. Evaluation focuses on readiness for discharge, understanding of medication regimen, and support resources. Structured tools like the teach-back method and standardized discharge checklists verify preparedness.

Post-discharge phone calls or telehealth visits within seven days, recommended by quality-measure frameworks, provide early feedback on symptom control and medication tolerance. When evaluation reveals confusion or barriers—financial constraints, transportation, or limited health literacy—nurses coordinate community resources to modify the plan accordingly.

Leadership in Evaluation

Board-certified nurses often lead unit-based evaluation initiatives. They chair morbidity-review meetings, mentor colleagues in data interpretation, and design improvement projects. Leadership involves translating individual evaluations into system learning. By presenting aggregated findings—such as patterns of catheter-related infection—they advocate for structural changes that enhance safety across populations.

Closing the Loop

Evaluation culminates in modification, completing the cyclical nature of the nursing process. Lessons drawn from one patient's course inform the next plan of care, progressively refining practice standards. The outcome is adaptive competence: the ability to maintain quality in the face of changing evidence, technology, and patient expectations.

The Science of Outcome Evaluation

Evaluation at the advanced-practice level combines clinical observation with outcome science. Every nursing intervention becomes a measurable hypothesis: if executed correctly, it should yield predictable physiologic and psychosocial results. Certified nurses therefore design evaluation plans at the moment of implementation, defining indicators, timelines, and benchmarks. Indicators include physiologic metrics—blood-pressure stability, oxygen consumption, weight trends—as well as functional measures such as six-minute-walk distance or return-to-work status.

Reliability and validity guide data selection. A reproducible measurement—daily weight using the same scale at the same time—ensures accuracy; a valid measurement truly reflects volume status rather than unrelated fluctuations. Awareness of measurement error prevents misinterpretation and inappropriate modification.

Data-Driven Clinical Judgement

Advanced evaluation transforms bedside observations into analytic reasoning. Nurses collate laboratory values, imaging reports, and patient narratives, constructing trend tables or dashboards. Data visualization clarifies patterns otherwise hidden in textual notes. A rising creatinine following diuretic escalation, coupled with unchanged pulmonary findings, prompts recalibration toward renal protection.

Benchmarking against institutional and national standards situates individual results within context. When a unit's post-angioplasty bleeding rate exceeds benchmark, nurses investigate procedural variables and re-educate staff on sheath removal technique. Continuous comparison transforms isolated evaluation into system improvement.

Advanced Use of Technology in Evaluation

Digital health records integrate algorithmic alerts that identify deviation from expected recovery trajectories. The expert nurse configures thresholds sensibly, avoiding alarm fatigue by tailoring parameters to individual baselines. Remote-monitoring platforms transmit biometric data—weight, heart rate, rhythm strips—directly into dashboards. Nurses interpret these in near real time, initiating early outreach when deviations appear.

Artificial-intelligence modules increasingly contribute predictive analytics; however, the human nurse interprets context. A prediction of "high risk for readmission" gains meaning only when reconciled with patient motivation, family support, and environmental factors. Judgment remains the decisive element of evaluation.

Multilevel Evaluation: Individual, Team, and System

Evaluation occurs on three interdependent levels.

Individual Patient Level: Focused on clinical outcomes and satisfaction. Tools such as the Kansas City Cardiomyopathy Questionnaire quantify perceived quality of life. The nurse correlates subjective scores with objective progress, validating improvement.

Team Level: Measures collaboration efficiency—timeliness of response, adherence to care pathways, and communication quality. Post-event debriefings identify lapses and reinforce effective behaviors.

System Level: Encompasses quality-improvement metrics—readmission rates, length of stay, cost of care. Nurses translate aggregate data into actionable policy proposals.

Integration across these levels ensures that micro-level evaluations feed macro-level change.

Modification Through Adaptive Learning

Modification is the creative response to evaluation findings. It requires flexibility without loss of rigor. When outcomes diverge from expectation, nurses dissect possible causes: intervention fidelity, patient adherence, or unforeseen comorbid factors. Plan adjustments follow a logic similar to the Plan-Do-Study-Act cycle—formulate modification, test on a small scale, evaluate effect, and disseminate successful change.

Adaptive learning uses feedback loops. For instance, introducing evening telehealth check-ins may reveal improved medication adherence; data confirming this success justify institutional adoption. Each loop closes knowledge gaps and refines care delivery.

Incorporating Patient-Generated Data

Wearable technology expands the scope of evaluation. Step counts, heart-rate variability, and sleep metrics provide longitudinal insight into functional recovery. Nurses verify device accuracy and teach patients to interpret outputs responsibly. When a sudden decline in daily steps coincides with elevated heart rate, early intervention prevents relapse.

Ethical evaluation requires consent for data use, clarity about storage, and education on privacy. Transparency sustains trust while leveraging innovation.

Evaluating Psychosocial Outcomes

Cardiovascular recovery intertwines with emotional and social adaptation. Nurses employ standardized tools—Hospital Anxiety and Depression Scale, Duke Activity Status Index—to quantify psychosocial dimensions. Repeated assessment across rehabilitation reveals trajectory rather than snapshot. When depression scores plateau despite physical improvement, modification introduces counseling or peer-support referral.

Social determinants are evaluated concurrently. Housing stability, access to nutrition, and family dynamics influence success. Addressing these through community linkage represents outcome-oriented compassion.

Research and Evidence Integration in Evaluation

Certified nurses contribute to the body of evidence by documenting and publishing evaluation findings. Participation in research strengthens methodological rigor. Understanding statistics—confidence intervals, p-values, effect sizes—empowers critical appraisal of new studies before integrating changes into practice. Evaluation thus bridges clinical service and scientific inquiry.

Leadership in Continuous Quality Improvement

Leadership transforms evaluation from a reactive audit to a proactive culture. Nurses chair quality councils, present dashboards, and coach peers in data interpretation. Transparent sharing of both achievements and failures encourages collective ownership. Recognition programs for evidence-based improvements reinforce motivation.

High-reliability principles—preoccupation with failure, sensitivity to operations, deference to expertise—frame leadership mindset. By fostering psychological safety, leaders invite reporting of near misses, converting potential harm into preventive knowledge.

Ethical and Legal Aspects of Modification

Evaluation and modification involve disclosure of results that may highlight errors. Ethical practice demands honesty tempered with constructive focus. Incident reporting protects patients and professionals when approached as learning rather than punishment.

Legal documentation follows institutional policy: factual, chronological, and devoid of judgmental language. When modification involves medication change or procedure adjustment, informed consent reflects the rationale and potential consequences. Maintaining transparency preserves trust and complies with regulatory standards.

Case Application: Evaluation Loop in Heart-Failure Management

An outpatient heart-failure program tracks weight, blood pressure, and self-reported symptoms daily. Analysis reveals that readmissions cluster among patients with limited literacy. Nurses modify educational materials to pictorial formats and conduct home visits. Subsequent evaluation shows a forty-percent reduction in readmissions. The cycle demonstrates how evidence-driven modification translates directly into measurable outcomes.

Personal Reflection and Professional Growth

Evaluation extends inward. Reflective journaling after complex cases cultivates insight into emotional reactions, decision bias, and resilience. Peer discussion groups encourage open examination of practice, reinforcing ethical accountability and continuous learning.

Chapter 4: Patient and Community Education

Education accounts for twenty-five percent of the certification examination and represents the outward expression of all prior domains. Knowledge gained through assessment, planning, and evaluation attains full value only when transmitted effectively to patients, families, and communities.

Principles of Adult Learning

Adult education is most effective when learners perceive relevance, draw on experience, and exercise autonomy. The cardiac-vascular nurse acts as facilitator rather than lecturer, engaging patients through dialogue and demonstration. Assessing readiness to learn prevents frustration and ensures timing aligns with emotional state and physical stamina. Immediately after an acute event, brief reassurance may suffice; deeper instruction follows stabilization.

Learning styles vary. Some patients benefit from printed material with diagrams; others prefer conversation or digital resources. The nurse tailors approach accordingly, confirming comprehension through return demonstration or verbalization. The goal is not rote recall but behavioral integration.

Health Literacy and Communication

Health-literacy assessment forms the foundation of effective education. Tools such as the Rapid Estimate of Adult Literacy in Medicine identify comprehension challenges. Nurses then simplify terminology—using "heart pump" instead of "ventricular contractility," or "water pill" for diuretic—without diminishing accuracy.

Language access is a matter of equity. Professional interpreters replace ad-hoc family translation to preserve accuracy and confidentiality. Written materials are provided in preferred language and reading level. Visual aids depicting portion sizes, fluid measurements, or symptom zones enhance clarity.

Communication extends to emotional literacy. Many patients equate cardiac disease with impending death. Sensitive discussion reframes the condition as manageable chronic illness, emphasizing control through adherence and lifestyle.

Core Education Topics in Cardiovascular Care

Medication Management – Understanding purpose, dosing, and potential side effects of each drug fosters adherence. Patients learn to organize schedules, avoid double-dosing, and recognize when to contact clinicians. Teaching includes safe storage and the importance of never discontinuing therapy abruptly.

Symptom Recognition – Early identification of decompensation—weight gain, swelling, increased dyspnea—prevents hospital readmission. The nurse provides individualized action plans specifying thresholds for calling the provider.

Dietary Instruction – Education integrates cultural preferences with nutritional science. Demonstrating label reading, sodium counting, and meal planning transforms abstract limits into daily practice. Collaborating with dietitians ensures consistency across the team.

Physical Activity – Using cardiac-rehabilitation frameworks, nurses teach safe progression from rest to structured exercise. Patients learn warm-up routines, intensity monitoring via Borg scale, and recovery practices.

Risk-Factor Modification – Smoking cessation, alcohol moderation, and stress management are addressed with motivational interviewing. Nurses assist in selecting realistic goals and connecting with support programs.

Behavioral-Change Strategies

Education succeeds when it triggers sustainable behavior change. The transtheoretical model—pre-contemplation through maintenance—guides tailored interventions. Nurses identify stage of readiness and provide appropriate support: information for contemplation, skill training for preparation, and reinforcement during maintenance.

Motivational interviewing enhances intrinsic motivation. Instead of instructing, the nurse explores ambivalence, elicits patient reasons for change, and reinforces self-efficacy. Statements such as "You've managed to walk twice this week despite fatigue" emphasize accomplishment and strengthen resolve.

Family and Caregiver Involvement

Cardiac-vascular outcomes depend heavily on family support. Nurses involve caregivers in every educational encounter, clarifying medication schedules, diet restrictions, and emergency actions. Family members learn signs of decompensation and communication channels for assistance. Education about caregiver self-care prevents burnout and maintains continuity.

Family meetings encourage shared decision-making for complex choices such as advanced therapies or end-of-life care. Transparent discussion fosters trust and alignment of expectations.

Community-Level Education

Beyond individual teaching, certified nurses influence population health through outreach programs. Screenings for hypertension, cholesterol, and diabetes detect risk early. Public seminars on diet and exercise translate clinical knowledge into community empowerment. Collaboration with schools, workplaces, and faith organizations extends reach to diverse demographics.

Community partnerships multiply impact. Working with local grocery stores to label heart-healthy options or organizing walking clubs converts abstract advice into accessible action. Nurses serve as advocates linking medical systems with public infrastructure.

Technology-Enhanced Education

Digital platforms amplify educational access. Mobile applications track medication adherence, activity, and blood-pressure readings, providing instant feedback. Nurses interpret data trends and adjust guidance accordingly. Online modules supplement in-person sessions, allowing review at the learner's pace.

Virtual support groups create peer connection and reduce isolation. Moderated forums ensure accurate information and emotional reinforcement. While leveraging technology, nurses uphold privacy through secure channels and consent procedures.

Cultural Competence in Education

Cultural competence requires awareness of one's own assumptions and genuine curiosity about others' beliefs. Nurses explore dietary customs, health rituals, and family decision structures. For instance, in cultures where elders hold authority, involving them in teaching sessions ensures acceptance. In communities valuing holistic medicine, nurses discuss how prescribed treatments coexist with traditional practices, identifying safe combinations and avoiding harmful interactions.

Cultural humility replaces presumption with partnership. Continuous learning and respectful questioning cultivate trust, allowing education to resonate authentically.

Evaluation of Educational Outcomes

Teaching effectiveness is measured through behavior, not just recollection. Follow-up assessments examine whether patients weigh themselves daily, maintain exercise logs, and achieve target blood-pressure control. When objectives remain unmet, nurses analyze barriers—complex regimen, limited finances, or misunderstanding—and modify strategy.

Peer review and mentorship sustain quality. Sharing successful methods during staff meetings or quality councils diffuses best practices throughout the organization.

Long-Term Self-Management Frameworks

Sustainable cardiovascular health depends on structured self-management. The nurse's task extends from initial teaching to cultivation of lifelong habits. Frameworks such as the Chronic Care Model emphasize informed patients, proactive teams, and supportive systems. Nurses coordinate with primary-care providers to establish scheduled follow-ups, remote monitoring, and community resources.

Daily self-management behaviors form the foundation: medication adherence, weight and symptom tracking, balanced nutrition, and scheduled activity. Nurses teach patients to interpret their own data—recognizing that a two-pound overnight weight gain signals fluid retention requiring action. Empowerment transforms compliance into partnership; patients become collaborators maintaining their own stability.

Reinforcement and Follow-Up

Education requires reinforcement to endure. Scheduled reinforcement at one week, one month, and three months after discharge maintains momentum. Each interaction reassesses understanding, celebrates successes, and addresses new barriers. For example, a patient who initially mastered sodium control may now struggle with medication affordability. Identifying evolving obstacles keeps interventions relevant.

Follow-up may occur in person or via telehealth. Video consultations allow observation of home environments—medication organization, dietary patterns, or exercise spaces—offering context for guidance. Nurses use motivational language to highlight progress while recalibrating goals.

Advocacy and Policy Education

Cardiac-vascular nurses extend education into advocacy, shaping environments that support health. They participate in policy initiatives promoting smoke-free spaces, community fitness infrastructure, and accessible blood-pressure screening. By translating bedside experiences into policy recommendations, nurses influence determinants of cardiovascular risk on a population level.

Educational outreach within professional organizations advances standards of care. Presenting outcomes of community programs at conferences fosters replication elsewhere. Mentoring novice nurses in patient education ensures continuity of expertise.

Addressing Social Determinants of Health

Effective education cannot ignore economic and social realities. Nurses assess transportation, food security, and financial capacity. When limited access to fresh produce threatens dietary adherence, collaboration with community food programs or mobile markets provides tangible solutions. Linking patients with social workers or financial counselors integrates clinical and social care.

Health inequities rooted in systemic barriers require advocacy at institutional levels. Culturally responsive outreach programs, bilingual staff recruitment, and inclusive educational materials reduce disparities. Nurses champion equity not as an adjunct but as central to patient education.

End-of-Life and Palliative Education

Advanced cardiac disease may progress despite optimal management. Education then shifts toward symptom control, comfort, and quality of life. Nurses explain palliative options, dispel misconceptions about withdrawal of care, and support families through decision-making. Discussions emphasize dignity, aligning interventions with patient values.

Teaching focuses on recognizing distress—dyspnea, fatigue, anxiety—and employing pharmacologic and non-pharmacologic relief. Families learn positioning techniques, relaxation strategies, and medication administration. Honest, compassionate dialogue replaces fear with understanding.

Community Partnerships and Outreach Models

Community partnerships transform individual education into collective prevention. Collaboration with local health departments establishes screening stations in community centers, workplaces, and schools. Data from these initiatives guide targeted interventions—blood-pressure-control campaigns in neighborhoods with high prevalence, or culturally tailored nutrition workshops.

Faith-based and civic organizations offer trusted platforms for dissemination. Nurses deliver sessions after worship services or community meetings, integrating messages with cultural values. Evaluation metrics—number of participants screened, referral completion rates—demonstrate impact and attract funding for program expansion.

School-Based Cardiovascular Education

Prevention begins early. Partnering with educators, nurses design age-appropriate curricula on nutrition, exercise, and stress management. Interactive demonstrations—measuring pulse before and after activity, comparing salt content of snacks—embed concepts experientially. Educating youth creates generational ripple effects as children influence family behaviors.

Workplace Wellness Programs

Cardiac-vascular nurses serve as consultants for workplace wellness initiatives. They assist employers in designing hypertension-screening days, ergonomic assessments, and physical-activity challenges. Education addresses sedentary risk and encourages micro-breaks for movement. Evaluating biometric outcomes over time validates program success and secures continued investment.

Integrating Technology for Population Education

Population-level digital education harnesses social media, webinars, and apps. Nurses develop content that balances accuracy with accessibility—short videos on blood-pressure measurement technique, infographics summarizing heart-healthy diets, or interactive quizzes reinforcing medication adherence.

Analytics from digital platforms guide refinement. Engagement rates reveal which messages resonate; feedback shapes future content. Maintaining professionalism online, nurses cite evidence without disclosing personal clinical details, preserving trust.

Measuring Community Education Outcomes

Community education evaluation mirrors clinical quality assurance. Metrics include screening numbers, referral uptake, behavioral changes, and reduced emergency visits. Surveys assess knowledge retention and satisfaction. Data inform grant proposals and policy advocacy. Reporting outcomes transparently enhances credibility and ensures accountability.

Leadership and Mentorship in Education

Certified nurses function as leaders, mentoring peers in teaching methodology and content accuracy. They conduct workshops on communication skills, cultural humility, and use of educational technology. Mentorship fosters a culture of continuous learning within healthcare organizations.

Leadership extends to curriculum design for orientation and continuing education programs. By embedding cardiovascular teaching into organizational training, nurses ensure consistent messaging across disciplines.

Integrating Education Across the Care Continuum

Education is not a discrete event but a continuum. From the first emergency encounter to long-term community support, nurses maintain coherent messaging. Consistent terminology across settings prevents confusion. For example, using identical color-coded symptom zones—green for stable, yellow for caution, red for emergency—simplifies patient understanding.

Transition-of-care communication includes handoff of educational achievements and pending goals. Receiving teams build on previous teaching rather than duplicating effort. This seamless continuity demonstrates professional collaboration and enhances outcomes.

Ethical Considerations in Education

Education carries ethical obligations: veracity, respect, and non-maleficence. Nurses ensure information accuracy, disclose limitations of knowledge, and avoid coercion. Teaching must respect autonomy; patients choose which changes to adopt. When cultural or personal beliefs conflict with recommendations, nurses negotiate feasible compromises that preserve dignity.

Documentation of education provided and patient responses serves both legal and ethical purposes. Accurate recording proves that informed consent and shared decision-making occurred.

Case Example – Community-Wide Hypertension Initiative

A regional hospital identifies high readmission rates for uncontrolled hypertension. Cardiac-vascular nurses lead a community initiative offering free screenings and group education sessions at local markets. Participants learn accurate home measurement techniques and dietary strategies. Follow-up clinics provide medication adjustment and reinforcement. After one year, average community systolic pressure decreases by eight mmHg, and hospital readmissions decline by twenty percent. This case illustrates how education extends the nurse's influence from bedside to population health.

Sustaining Motivation and Resilience

Behavioral maintenance requires sustained motivation. Nurses teach relapse-prevention strategies—anticipating triggers such as holidays or stress, and preparing adaptive responses. Encouraging self-forgiveness for occasional lapses prevents abandonment of progress. Celebrating incremental achievements reinforces commitment.

Peer-support networks further resilience. Group sessions allow participants to share challenges and solutions, normalizing struggle and promoting collective encouragement. The nurse acts as facilitator, maintaining focus and factual accuracy.

Integration with National Health Goals

Education aligns with broader public-health frameworks such as national objectives for cardiovascular disease reduction. Nurses translate these macro goals into micro actions: promoting blood-pressure screening, cholesterol management, and smoking cessation within their communities. Reporting outcomes contributes data to state and national registries, closing the loop between practice and policy.

Professional Growth Through Education

Teaching others refines the educator's own expertise. Preparing content necessitates review of current literature, reinforcing evidence familiarity. Reflection on learner feedback sharpens communication. Certified nurses document teaching hours and outcomes as part of continuing-education portfolios, demonstrating lifelong learning and accountability.

Frameworks for Lifelong Learning in Cardiac-Vascular Health

Education at the advanced level transcends episodic instruction and becomes a structured continuum. The expert nurse designs longitudinal learning plans that align with the patient's recovery phases—acute stabilization, rehabilitation, and lifelong maintenance. Each phase has its own objectives: immediate comprehension of discharge orders, skill acquisition during rehabilitation, and sustained self-efficacy after reintegration into daily life.

Learning plans are documented within the care record as living documents. Updates occur whenever therapy changes, new devices are implanted, or lifestyle challenges emerge. This dynamic approach ensures that education evolves with the patient's condition rather than remaining static handouts.

Cognitive and Behavioral Science Foundations

Neuroscientific insight into learning underpins advanced teaching. Repetition and multisensory engagement strengthen neural pathways; therefore, education combines verbal explanation, visual aids, and kinesthetic practice. Emotional salience enhances retention—linking new information to personal goals such as attending a grandchild's wedding transforms abstract instruction into motivation.

Behavioral economics contributes additional tools. "Nudge" strategies—placing medication organizers on breakfast tables, arranging clinic schedules that coincide with routine errands—reduce friction between intention and action. Understanding these subtle influences enables nurses to embed adherence into lifestyle.

Tailored Education for Special Populations

Cardiac-vascular care encompasses diverse populations requiring customized approaches.

Older adults benefit from slower pacing, larger print, and repetition to accommodate sensory changes. Reinforcing small successes preserves dignity and confidence.

Adolescents and young adults with congenital or early-onset disease need developmentally appropriate explanations emphasizing autonomy and technology integration. Transition programs from pediatric to adult care maintain continuity.

Patients with cognitive impairment require involvement of caregivers, simplified routines, and use of memory aids.

Culturally diverse populations necessitate adaptation to language, diet, and health beliefs. Collaborating with cultural mediators ensures authenticity and avoids stereotyping.

Interprofessional Education and Collaboration

Education does not occur in isolation. Dietitians, pharmacists, physical therapists, and social workers contribute domain-specific instruction. The cardiac-vascular nurse functions as integrator, ensuring consistent messages. Interprofessional education sessions for patients—where each specialist explains their role—demystify the care process and foster trust.

For healthcare teams, cross-training enhances consistency. Nurses lead in-service programs on accurate blood-pressure measurement, heart-failure self-management protocols, and motivational interviewing. Through teaching peers, they extend educational influence exponentially.

Community Empowerment and Health Promotion

Advanced education initiatives aim to alter community norms, not just individual behavior. Nurses organize "heart-health festivals" combining screenings, demonstrations, and interactive workshops. By partnering with local chefs to create low-sodium recipes or with gyms for subsidized memberships, education translates into community infrastructure.

Faith-based outreach remains powerful in many regions. Collaborating with clergy allows integration of health messages into sermons and congregational events. Trust inherent in these relationships amplifies acceptance of prevention messages.

Utilizing Mass Media and Social Platforms Responsibly

Modern education campaigns rely on media literacy. Nurses trained in communication craft clear, evidence-based messages for television, radio, and social media while avoiding sensationalism. Posts emphasize practical actions—checking blood pressure, recognizing stroke signs, moderating salt intake—paired with credible citations.

Interactive digital sessions via webinars or live streams enable question-and-answer engagement with large audiences. Recorded versions remain accessible for asynchronous learning, expanding reach to shift workers or rural residents.

Ethical digital presence requires verification of information sources, disclosure of affiliations, and respect for privacy. Nurses model professionalism online, countering misinformation with empathy rather than confrontation.

Technology-Enhanced Personalized Education

Wearable devices and patient portals revolutionize personalization. Nurses configure dashboards displaying blood-pressure trends, weight, and activity metrics, transforming data into teaching tools. Reviewing graphs together with patients converts abstract numbers into tangible stories of progress or relapse.

Gamification increases engagement: awarding virtual badges for consecutive days of medication adherence or steps walked reinforces consistency. Regular feedback loops, such as weekly automated summaries, sustain motivation.

However, digital equity remains a concern. Nurses identify barriers—lack of devices, internet access, or digital literacy—and connect patients with community resources to bridge gaps.

Measuring Educational Impact

At the advanced level, evaluation of education parallels research methodology. Outcome indicators include knowledge retention, behavioral change, clinical improvement, and quality-of-life enhancement. Pre- and post-tests quantify cognitive gains; follow-up surveys capture sustained behavior.

Qualitative evaluation—patient narratives, focus groups, and reflective interviews—reveals emotional resonance and unanticipated barriers. Integrating both quantitative and qualitative data provides a holistic picture of educational efficacy.

Statistical analysis within quality-improvement frameworks (for example, a 10 percent rise in patients meeting blood-pressure goals after a community campaign) demonstrates tangible return on educational investment.

Education in Crisis and Disaster Preparedness

During natural disasters or pandemics, continuity of cardiovascular care depends on rapid education. Nurses prepare emergency packets detailing medication lists, device information, and contact numbers. Teaching focuses on medication substitution if supply chains fail, safe sheltering for those dependent on electrical devices, and stress-management strategies to mitigate cardiovascular strain.

Community drills incorporate cardiovascular considerations—availability of defibrillators, triage of cardiac patients, and transportation plans for dialysis or infusion therapies. Post-crisis debriefing becomes another educational moment, reinforcing resilience and preparedness.

Ethics and Advocacy in Education

Ethical teaching honors truthfulness and cultural respect. When discussing prognosis or lifestyle limits, honesty is balanced with hope. Advocacy ensures that patients receive not only information but the means to act upon it—access to affordable medications, nutritious food, and safe environments for exercise.

At policy levels, nurses lobby for legislation mandating clear food labeling, sodium reduction in processed foods, and funding for community screening. Advocacy education empowers patients to engage politically, recognizing that structural change complements personal effort.

Global and Environmental Perspectives

Cardiovascular education now encompasses planetary health. Air pollution, climate-related heat stress, and food insecurity influence cardiac outcomes. Nurses educate communities about environmental stewardship—reducing exposure to pollutants, supporting sustainable agriculture, and recognizing climate-related symptoms such as dehydration-induced arrhythmia. Global collaboration through tele-education connects nurses worldwide, exchanging successful prevention strategies adaptable across cultures.

Building a Culture of Learning Within Healthcare Organizations

Within institutions, cardiac-vascular nurses establish continuous-learning cultures. Unit-based "learning huddles" allow quick dissemination of new evidence. Bulletin boards display simplified summaries of recent guidelines, turning hallways into learning spaces. Encouraging bedside teaching rounds where experienced nurses explain rationale to peers embeds education in workflow.

Recognition systems—continuing-education credits, certification support, and public acknowledgment—sustain enthusiasm. When education becomes an expected daily activity rather than an occasional event, knowledge remains current and morale high.

Case Example – Digital Rehabilitation Education Program

A hospital develops a hybrid cardiac-rehabilitation program integrating in-person sessions with an online platform. Nurses upload weekly exercise videos, nutrition modules, and interactive quizzes. Participants log progress and receive individualized feedback. Over six months, average adherence improves by thirty percent compared with traditional models. The project illustrates how advanced education leverages technology to extend reach while preserving human connection.

Reflection on the Evolving Educator Role

In the modern cardiovascular landscape, the nurse-educator embodies scientific literacy, cultural humility, and digital fluency. The educator's credibility derives from clinical competence and genuine empathy. Every conversation, from bedside teaching to public advocacy, becomes an opportunity to reduce disease burden and inspire autonomy.

By merging compassion with data-driven strategy, the cardiac-vascular nurse transforms education into a public-health intervention. Through persistent dialogue, tailored resources, and equitable access, these professionals cultivate communities that not only survive cardiovascular disease but thrive beyond it.

Chapter-5: Practice Questions

Question (1-100)

Q1. A patient with acute left-sided heart failure presents with severe dyspnea, crackles on auscultation, and pink frothy sputum. Which underlying mechanism most directly explains these findings?

(A) Decreased systemic vascular resistance
(B) Reduced preload from hypovolemia
(C) Increased oncotic pressure in alveoli
(D) Increased pulmonary capillary hydrostatic pressure

Q2. A postoperative cardiac surgery patient develops a sudden drop in blood pressure and muffled heart sounds with jugular venous distension. What is the most likely cause?

(A) Pulmonary embolism
(B) Hypovolemic shock
(C) Cardiac tamponade
(D) Anaphylaxis

Q3. A patient with atrial fibrillation is at greatest risk for which complication?

(A) Thromboembolic stroke
(B) Cardiac hypertrophy
(C) Pulmonary hypertension
(D) Ventricular septal rupture

Q4. A patient receiving intravenous heparin develops a platelet count drop from 300,000/µL to 90,000/µL within five days. What is the priority action?

(A) Discontinue heparin immediately
(B) Continue therapy and recheck in 24 hours
(C) Increase the heparin dose
(D) Administer vitamin K

Q5. During assessment of a patient with intermittent claudication, which finding is most characteristic?

(A) Leg pain relieved by rest
(B) Bilateral leg edema
(C) Constant burning foot pain
(D) Leg pain relieved by elevation

Q6. A patient with cardiogenic shock has a blood pressure of 80/50 mmHg and cold clammy skin. What is the primary physiologic disturbance?

(A) Hypervolemia
(B) Decreased cardiac output
(C) Reduced afterload
(D) Increased preload

Q7. Which laboratory value is most specific for diagnosing myocardial infarction?

(A) Elevated myoglobin
(B) Elevated CK-MB
(C) Elevated BNP
(D) Elevated troponin I

Q8. A patient with chronic heart failure reports gaining 3 pounds in two days. What does this most likely indicate?

(A) Improved cardiac function
(B) Dehydration
(C) Muscle hypertrophy
(D) Fluid retention

Q9. A nurse notes tall peaked T waves on an ECG. Which electrolyte imbalance is most likely present?

(A) Hypokalemia
(B) Hyponatremia
(C) Hyperkalemia
(D) Hypocalcemia

Q10. A patient experiences chest pain that is relieved by nitroglycerin. What is the most likely mechanism of action?

(A) Coronary artery vasoconstriction
(B) Venodilation reducing preload
(C) Increased myocardial oxygen demand
(D) Increased heart rate

Q11. A patient recovering from CABG surgery has 300 mL chest tube output in one hour. What is the priority action?

(A) Document and continue monitoring
(B) Clamp the chest tube
(C) Elevate the head of bed
(D) Notify the surgeon immediately

Q12. Which finding indicates right-sided heart failure?

(A) Peripheral edema
(B) Pulmonary crackles
(C) Orthopnea
(D) Hemoptysis

Q13. A patient with severe aortic stenosis reports syncope during exertion. What is the primary cause?

(A) Reduced cerebral perfusion
(B) Increased coronary perfusion
(C) Hypervolemia

(D) Bradycardia

Q14. A patient receiving warfarin has an INR of 5.5 without bleeding. What is the appropriate intervention?

(A) Begin heparin therapy
(B) Hold the next dose
(C) Administer additional warfarin
(D) Increase vitamin K intake drastically

Q15. A patient develops sudden unilateral leg swelling and pain. What is the most likely diagnosis?

(A) Lymphedema
(B) Deep vein thrombosis
(C) Arterial occlusion
(D) Cellulitis

Q16. A patient in ventricular fibrillation requires immediate intervention. What is the first action?

(A) Defibrillate
(B) Begin chest compressions
(C) Administer atropine
(D) Give amiodarone

Q17. Which symptom is most typical of chronic venous insufficiency?

(A) Cool pale extremities
(B) Brownish skin discoloration
(C) Intermittent claudication
(D) Absent pedal pulses

Q18. A patient with pulmonary embolism most commonly presents with which symptom?

(A) Bradycardia
(B) Sudden dyspnea
(C) Hypertension
(D) Hyperglycemia

Q19. Which intervention reduces the risk of ventilator-associated pneumonia?

(A) Supine positioning
(B) Delaying extubation
(C) Routine sedation interruption
(D) Limiting oral care

Q20. A patient with hypertensive crisis has BP 220/120 mmHg and headache. What is the immediate goal of therapy?

(A) Normalize blood pressure within 30 minutes
(B) Administer oral diuretics only
(C) Increase heart rate
(D) Reduce BP gradually to prevent organ damage

Q21. A patient with inferior wall myocardial infarction develops hypotension and clear lung sounds. Which complication is most likely present?

(A) Acute mitral regurgitation
(B) Ventricular septal rupture
(C) Left ventricular failure
(D) Right ventricular infarction

Q22. A patient with chronic hypertension develops left ventricular hypertrophy. What is the primary adaptive mechanism involved?

(A) Increased chamber dilation
(B) Valve leaflet calcification
(C) Reduced contractility
(D) Myocardial fiber thickening

Q23. A patient reports crushing substernal chest pain radiating to the left arm lasting 40 minutes. What is the most appropriate initial diagnostic test?

(A) 12-lead ECG
(B) Echocardiogram
(C) Cardiac MRI
(D) Chest X-ray

Q24. A postoperative patient becomes restless and confused with oxygen saturation of 86%. What is the priority nursing action?

(A) Reassure the patient only
(B) Provide oral fluids
(C) Administer supplemental oxygen
(D) Document findings

Q25. A patient with mitral valve stenosis is most likely to develop which complication?

(A) Pulmonary congestion
(B) Aortic aneurysm
(C) Systemic hypertension
(D) Bradycardia

Q26. Which assessment finding is most indicative of decreased cardiac output?

(A) Bounding peripheral pulses
(B) Warm flushed skin
(C) Elevated temperature
(D) Decreased urine output

Q27. A patient with pericarditis reports chest pain that improves when leaning forward. What is the underlying cause of pain relief?

(A) Reduced myocardial oxygen demand
(B) Improved pulmonary expansion
(C) Increased coronary perfusion

(D) Decreased pericardial friction

Q28. A patient receiving digoxin presents with nausea and visual halos. What is the most likely explanation?

(A) Therapeutic effect
(B) Drug toxicity
(C) Hypoglycemia
(D) Allergic reaction

Q29. Which intervention is most effective in preventing deep vein thrombosis in immobilized patients?

(A) Sequential compression devices
(B) Limiting fluid intake
(C) Bed rest
(D) Leg elevation only

Q30. A patient with heart failure is prescribed an ACE inhibitor. What is the primary therapeutic effect?

(A) Increased heart rate
(B) Increased sodium retention
(C) Decreased renal perfusion
(D) Reduced afterload

Q31. A patient with acute pulmonary edema is most likely to exhibit which finding?

(A) Pink frothy sputum
(B) Dry cough
(C) Slow respirations
(D) Absent breath sounds

Q32. A patient develops sudden chest pain and unequal blood pressures in both arms. What condition should be suspected?

(A) Stable angina
(B) Aortic dissection
(C) Pericardial effusion
(D) Myocardial infarction

Q33. Which ECG change is characteristic of hypokalemia?

(A) ST elevation
(B) Wide QRS complex
(C) Peaked T waves
(D) Prolonged QT interval

Q34. A patient with cardiomyopathy has an ejection fraction of 25%. What does this indicate?

(A) Adequate preload
(B) Hyperdynamic circulation
(C) Normal ventricular function
(D) Severe systolic dysfunction

Q35. A patient experiences syncope after standing quickly. What is the most likely cause?

(A) Hypervolemia
(B) Hypertensive crisis
(C) Orthostatic hypotension
(D) Pulmonary edema

Q36. A patient with bacterial endocarditis is at risk for which complication?

(A) Osteoporosis
(B) Renal stones
(C) Stroke from emboli
(D) Hypoglycemia

Q37. Which symptom is most consistent with stable angina?

(A) Pain at rest lasting hours
(B) Sudden tearing chest pain
(C) Constant chest tenderness
(D) Pain triggered by exertion and relieved by rest

Q38. A patient with chronic atrial fibrillation is prescribed anticoagulation primarily to prevent which outcome?

(A) Bradycardia
(B) Valve calcification
(C) Systemic embolization
(D) Ventricular hypertrophy

Q39. A patient with severe anemia has a hemoglobin of 6 g/dL. How does this affect cardiac workload?

(A) Decreases myocardial oxygen demand
(B) Increases cardiac output demand
(C) Reduces heart rate
(D) Causes vasoconstriction only

Q40. A patient with hypertrophic cardiomyopathy experiences sudden cardiac arrest. What is a common underlying mechanism?

(A) Hypoglycemia
(B) Renal failure
(C) Pulmonary infection
(D) Ventricular arrhythmia

Q41. A patient with acute coronary syndrome is given aspirin upon arrival to the emergency department. What is the primary reason for this intervention?

(A) Dissolve existing clot
(B) Inhibit platelet aggregation

(C) Lower blood pressure
(D) Reduce heart rate

Q42. A patient with chronic heart failure has elevated BNP levels. What does this indicate?
(A) Improved ventricular function
(B) Ventricular wall stretch
(C) Dehydration
(D) Decreased preload

Q43. A patient presents with sudden onset of severe chest pain radiating to the back and a widened mediastinum on chest X-ray. What is the most likely diagnosis?
(A) Gastroesophageal reflux
(B) Stable angina
(C) Aortic dissection
(D) Pulmonary embolism

Q44. A patient with second-degree type II atrioventricular block is most at risk for which complication?
(A) Complete heart block
(B) Hypertensive crisis
(C) Pulmonary edema
(D) Atrial fibrillation

Q45. A patient with peripheral arterial disease reports rest pain in the toes that worsens at night. What does this indicate?
(A) Venous insufficiency
(B) Cellulitis
(C) Improved collateral circulation
(D) Critical limb ischemia

Q46. A patient develops hypotension after rapid removal of 2 liters of pericardial fluid. What is the likely cause?
(A) Acute vasodilation
(B) Renal failure
(C) Reperfusion injury
(D) Myocardial rupture

Q47. A patient with atrial flutter has a ventricular rate of 150 beats per minute. What is the typical atrial rate in this rhythm?
(A) 300 beats per minute
(B) 100 beats per minute
(C) 60 beats per minute
(D) 150 beats per minute

Q48. A patient with acute decompensated heart failure is prescribed intravenous furosemide. What is the expected effect?
(A) Decreased urine output
(B) Reduced preload
(C) Increased afterload
(D) Increased fluid retention

Q49. A patient experiences chest pain during exercise that resolves within five minutes of rest. What is the underlying pathology?
(A) Complete coronary occlusion
(B) Transient myocardial ischemia
(C) Coronary artery spasm only
(D) Plaque rupture

Q50. A patient with severe hyperkalemia develops a widened QRS complex. What is the priority treatment?
(A) Initiate dialysis immediately
(B) Administer calcium gluconate
(C) Provide oral potassium supplements
(D) Give insulin with glucose

Q51. A patient with infective endocarditis develops hematuria and flank pain. What is the most likely cause?
(A) Renal embolism
(B) Dehydration
(C) Nephrolithiasis
(D) Urinary tract infection

Q52. A patient with heart failure has an S3 heart sound. What does this indicate?
(A) Pericardial friction
(B) Increased ventricular compliance
(C) Rapid ventricular filling
(D) Valve stenosis

Q53. A patient with a mechanical heart valve requires long-term therapy to prevent which complication?
(A) Hypertension
(B) Thrombus formation
(C) Myocardial hypertrophy
(D) Valve stenosis

Q54. A patient develops sudden shortness of breath after a long flight. What is the most likely diagnosis?
(A) Pneumothorax
(B) Pulmonary embolism
(C) Asthma exacerbation
(D) Heart block

Q55. A patient with cardiogenic shock is receiving an inotropic agent. What is the primary goal of this therapy?
(A) Decrease heart rate

(B) Reduce blood volume
(C) Induce vasoconstriction only
(D) Increase myocardial contractility

Q56. A patient with hypertension is advised to reduce sodium intake. What is the main rationale?
(A) Increase potassium excretion
(B) Reduce fluid retention
(C) Enhance glucose metabolism
(D) Decrease heart rate

Q57. A patient experiences palpitations and dizziness with a heart rate of 180 beats per minute and narrow QRS complexes. What rhythm is most likely present?
(A) Sinus bradycardia
(B) Complete heart block
(C) Supraventricular tachycardia
(D) Ventricular tachycardia

Q58. A patient with chronic kidney disease is at increased risk for which electrolyte imbalance affecting the heart?
(A) Hypokalemia
(B) Hypernatremia
(C) Hyperkalemia
(D) Hypocalcemia

Q59. A patient with acute myocardial infarction develops sudden papillary muscle dysfunction. What complication may result?
(A) Aortic stenosis
(B) Tricuspid atresia
(C) Pulmonary stenosis
(D) Mitral regurgitation

Q60. A patient in shock has a lactate level of 6 mmol/L. What does this indicate?
(A) Adequate perfusion
(B) Normal metabolism
(C) Tissue hypoxia
(D) Improved oxygenation

Q61. A 64-year-old male with history of hypertension presents with sudden crushing chest pain, diaphoresis, and ST elevation in leads II, III, and aVF. Blood pressure is 88/60 mmHg with clear lung fields. Which immediate intervention is most appropriate?
(A) Initiate rapid normal saline bolus
(B) Start high-dose beta-blocker
(C) Administer intravenous nitroglycerin infusion
(D) Give intravenous diuretic

Q62. A patient two days post-CABG develops sudden dyspnea, tachycardia, and decreased oxygen saturation. Chest tube output has been minimal. What is the most likely cause?
(A) Pneumonia
(B) Pericardial tamponade
(C) Atelectasis
(D) Pulmonary embolism

Q63. A patient with chronic heart failure forgets to take prescribed diuretics for three days and presents with weight gain, edema, and orthopnea. What is the priority nursing action?
(A) Begin chest physiotherapy
(B) Restrict oxygen therapy
(C) Encourage increased fluid intake
(D) Administer prescribed IV diuretic

Q64. A patient receiving warfarin for atrial fibrillation presents with sudden severe headache and an INR of 6.2. What is the priority intervention?
(A) Encourage ambulation
(B) Provide iron supplements
(C) Continue same dose
(D) Administer vitamin K

Q65. A patient with sepsis develops hypotension despite adequate fluid resuscitation and shows elevated cardiac filling pressures with low cardiac output. What type of shock is developing?
(A) Cardiogenic shock
(B) Neurogenic shock
(C) Distributive shock
(D) Hypovolemic shock

Q66. A patient with hypertrophic cardiomyopathy collapses during exercise. Which intervention is most likely to prevent recurrence?
(A) Long-term oxygen therapy
(B) Fluid restriction
(C) Implantable cardioverter-defibrillator placement
(D) Routine aspirin therapy

Q67. A 70-year-old with severe aortic stenosis develops chest pain and syncope during minimal exertion. What is the definitive treatment?

(A) Beta-blocker therapy only
(B) Balloon angioplasty
(C) Aortic valve replacement
(D) Diuretic therapy

Q68. A patient receiving IV amiodarone develops bradycardia and hypotension. What is the most appropriate action?
(A) Discontinue infusion temporarily
(B) Administer potassium
(C) Encourage ambulation
(D) Increase infusion rate

Q69. A patient presents with tearing chest pain radiating to the back and unequal pulses in upper extremities. Blood pressure is 210/110 mmHg. What is the priority management?
(A) Rapid blood pressure reduction with IV antihypertensive
(B) Administer diuretics only
(C) Immediate thrombolysis
(D) Encourage deep breathing exercises

Q70. A patient with chronic atrial fibrillation suddenly develops slurred speech and right-sided weakness. What is the most likely cause?
(A) Hypertensive crisis
(B) Systemic embolization to cerebral artery
(C) Anxiety attack
(D) Hypoglycemia

Q71. A patient post-myocardial infarction develops a new loud systolic murmur and pulmonary edema. What mechanical complication is most likely?
(A) First-degree AV block
(B) Sinus bradycardia
(C) Ventricular septal rupture
(D) Pericarditis

Q72. A patient with acute pulmonary embolism is hypotensive and tachycardic. What is the most appropriate initial therapy?
(A) Administer beta-blocker
(B) Thrombolytic therapy
(C) Encourage ambulation
(D) Oral anticoagulation only

Q73. A patient with heart failure has potassium level of 2.8 mEq/L after aggressive diuresis. What complication is most concerning?
(A) Hypertension
(B) Ventricular arrhythmia
(C) Hyperglycemia
(D) Bradycardia

Q74. A patient presents with crushing chest pain but normal troponin levels initially. What should be done next?
(A) Repeat troponin in several hours
(B) Discharge immediately
(C) Ignore symptoms
(D) Prescribe antibiotics

Q75. A patient with severe mitral regurgitation develops worsening dyspnea and fatigue. What is the primary hemodynamic effect?
(A) Decreased left atrial size
(B) Volume overload of left atrium
(C) Reduced pulmonary pressure
(D) Increased forward stroke volume

Q76. A patient with infective endocarditis is scheduled for dental extraction. What is the key preventive measure?
(A) Stop anticoagulation permanently
(B) Administer prophylactic antibiotics
(C) Withhold antibiotics
(D) Restrict fluids

Q77. A patient in ventricular tachycardia with a pulse is hypotensive and altered. What is the priority intervention?
(A) Encourage coughing
(B) Observation only
(C) Immediate synchronized cardioversion
(D) Oral medication administration

Q78. A patient with chronic venous insufficiency develops a shallow ulcer near the medial ankle. What is the most appropriate initial management?
(A) Elevate leg only
(B) Cold compress application
(C) Apply compression therapy
(D) Surgical amputation

Q79. A patient with acute coronary syndrome develops sudden bradycardia and hypotension after inferior MI. What is the likely cause?
(A) Hyperkalemia
(B) Fluid overload
(C) Increased sympathetic tone
(D) Vagal stimulation

Q80. A patient with chronic heart failure is noncompliant with low-sodium diet and

presents with severe dyspnea and crackles. What is the primary pathophysiologic change?
(A) Reduced systemic resistance
(B) Decreased preload
(C) Increased fluid retention
(D) Increased myocardial oxygen supply

Q81. A 58-year-old patient with uncontrolled hypertension presents with sudden onset severe headache, blurred vision, and blood pressure of 230/120 mmHg. Fundoscopic exam shows papilledema. What is the priority management?
(A) Immediate rapid normalization of blood pressure
(B) Controlled IV antihypertensive infusion
(C) Oral diuretic therapy only
(D) Observation for 24 hours

Q82. A patient with anterior wall myocardial infarction develops acute shortness of breath and bilateral crackles. Blood pressure is 90/60 mmHg. What complication is most likely?
(A) Pericarditis
(B) Aortic stenosis
(C) Acute left ventricular failure
(D) Right ventricular infarction

Q83. A patient receiving thrombolytic therapy for STEMI develops gum bleeding and oozing from IV sites. What is the appropriate nursing action?
(A) Apply heat packs
(B) Stop infusion and notify provider
(C) Continue infusion at same rate
(D) Encourage ambulation

Q84. A patient with dilated cardiomyopathy has progressive fatigue and reduced exercise tolerance. Echocardiogram shows EF 30%. What medication class improves survival?
(A) Calcium supplements
(B) ACE inhibitors
(C) NSAIDs
(D) Antacids

Q85. A patient develops sudden chest pain and hypotension after central line placement. Breath sounds are absent on the right side. What is the most likely cause?
(A) Tension pneumothorax
(B) Bronchitis
(C) Pulmonary edema
(D) Myocardial infarction

Q86. A patient with chronic atrial fibrillation presents with rapid ventricular response at 160 bpm and hypotension. What is the priority intervention?
(A) Immediate synchronized cardioversion
(B) Oral anticoagulation
(C) Encourage rest
(D) Administer diuretic

Q87. A patient with peripheral arterial disease reports a non-healing ulcer on the toe with pale surrounding skin. What is the underlying mechanism?
(A) Arterial insufficiency
(B) Lymphatic obstruction
(C) Fungal infection
(D) Venous hypertension

Q88. A patient with heart failure is taking spironolactone and develops muscle weakness with potassium level 6.1 mEq/L. What is the likely cause?
(A) Hyperkalemia from potassium-sparing effect
(B) Hypokalemia
(C) Hypoglycemia
(D) Dehydration

Q89. A patient post-cardiac catheterization develops swelling and bruit at the insertion site. What complication is suspected?
(A) Cellulitis
(B) Hematoma
(C) Pseudoaneurysm
(D) Lymphedema

Q90. A patient with infective endocarditis suddenly develops left-sided weakness. What is the immediate concern?
(A) Hyperglycemia
(B) Cerebral embolism
(C) Hypotension
(D) Electrolyte imbalance

Q91. A patient with cardiogenic shock has cool extremities and decreased urine output. Which parameter best indicates improvement?
(A) Rising lactate levels
(B) Increasing urine output
(C) Persistent hypotension
(D) Worsening confusion

Q92. A patient with unstable angina reports chest pain at rest lasting 15 minutes. Troponin

levels are normal. What is the appropriate management?
(A) Discharge home
(B) Prescribe antibiotics
(C) Initiate antiplatelet and anticoagulant therapy
(D) Provide only pain medication

Q93. A patient with severe anemia and coronary artery disease develops chest pain. What is the precipitating factor?
(A) Reduced oxygen-carrying capacity
(B) Increased oxygen delivery
(C) Decreased heart rate
(D) Fluid overload

Q94. A patient with long-standing hypertension develops chronic kidney disease. What is the pathophysiologic link?
(A) Increased insulin production
(B) Decreased renal perfusion from vascular damage
(C) Enhanced filtration capacity
(D) Reduced sodium retention

Q95. A patient develops sudden severe dyspnea and pink frothy sputum after myocardial infarction. What is the immediate intervention?
(A) Administer high-flow oxygen and diuretics
(B) Provide oral fluids
(C) Lay patient flat
(D) Encourage ambulation

Q96. A patient with atrial fibrillation is scheduled for elective cardioversion. What is required beforehand if arrhythmia duration exceeds 48 hours?
(A) Immediate pacing
(B) Anticoagulation for several weeks
(C) Fluid restriction
(D) No preparation needed

Q97. A patient with severe sepsis develops warm flushed skin and bounding pulses. What stage of shock is this?
(A) Early distributive
(B) Obstructive
(C) Hypovolemic
(D) Late cardiogenic

Q98. A patient with pulmonary hypertension complains of increasing fatigue and edema. What is the primary cardiac effect?
(A) Aortic dilation
(B) Mitral stenosis
(C) Left ventricular hypertrophy
(D) Right ventricular strain

Q99. A patient post-angioplasty develops chest pain and ST elevation again. What is the most likely cause?
(A) Restenosis or acute re-occlusion
(B) Anxiety
(C) Dehydration
(D) Pneumonia

Q100. A patient with chronic heart failure presents with confusion and cool extremities. Blood pressure is 78/50 mmHg. What is the most likely condition?
(A) Cardiogenic shock
(B) Controlled hypertension
(C) Stable angina
(D) Hypervolemia

Answer Key and Explanation (1-100)

Q1. Answer: D

Explanation: Acute left-sided heart failure leads to elevated pressure in the left atrium and pulmonary veins. This increases pulmonary capillary hydrostatic pressure, causing fluid to move into the alveolar spaces. The accumulation of fluid results in pulmonary edema, which manifests as crackles and pink frothy sputum. Dyspnea occurs due to impaired gas exchange across fluid-filled alveoli. The other mechanisms do not directly cause fluid transudation into the alveoli in this scenario.

Q2. Answer: C

Explanation: The combination of hypotension, muffled heart sounds, and jugular venous distension suggests cardiac tamponade. Fluid accumulation in the pericardial sac compresses the heart and restricts ventricular filling. This leads to decreased stroke volume and reduced cardiac output. As a result, systemic blood pressure falls and venous pressure rises. Prompt recognition is essential because untreated tamponade can rapidly become life-threatening.

Q3. Answer: A

Explanation: Atrial fibrillation causes ineffective atrial contraction, leading to blood stasis in the atria. Stagnant blood increases the risk of thrombus formation, especially in the left atrial appendage. If a clot dislodges, it may travel to cerebral circulation and cause an ischemic stroke. Anticoagulation therapy is often prescribed to reduce this risk. The other complications are not directly caused by atrial fibrillation.

Q4. Answer: A

Explanation: A significant drop in platelet count after heparin exposure suggests heparin-induced thrombocytopenia. This immune-mediated reaction increases the risk of thrombosis rather than bleeding. Immediate discontinuation of heparin is necessary to prevent further complications. Alternative anticoagulation may be required. Early identification reduces the risk of life-threatening clot formation.

Q5. Answer: A

Explanation: Intermittent claudication is caused by peripheral arterial disease leading to reduced blood flow during exertion. Pain typically occurs with activity due to increased oxygen demand in muscles. Rest decreases demand and relieves the pain. This pattern differentiates it from venous disorders where elevation may help. Edema and constant burning pain suggest different underlying conditions.

Q6. Answer: B

Explanation: Cardiogenic shock results from the heart's inability to pump effectively. Decreased cardiac output leads to hypotension and poor tissue perfusion. Compensatory vasoconstriction causes cold, clammy skin. Without prompt intervention, organ dysfunction may occur. The underlying issue is impaired myocardial contractility.

Q7. Answer: D

Explanation: Troponin I is highly specific for myocardial injury. It rises within hours after infarction and remains elevated for several days. This makes it a reliable marker for diagnosing myocardial infarction. Other markers may rise but are less specific. Troponin levels correlate with the extent of myocardial damage.

Q8. Answer: D

Explanation: Rapid weight gain in heart failure typically reflects fluid accumulation. Sodium and water retention occur due to decreased cardiac output and neurohormonal activation. Monitoring daily weight helps detect early decompensation. Early intervention can prevent hospitalization. Muscle growth does not occur this quickly.

Q9. Answer: C

Explanation: Hyperkalemia alters cardiac electrical activity and commonly produces peaked T waves. Elevated serum potassium affects myocardial repolarization. If untreated, it may progress to life-threatening arrhythmias. Early recognition allows timely treatment to stabilize the myocardium. Electrolyte monitoring is critical in cardiac patients.

Q10. Answer: B

Explanation: Nitroglycerin primarily causes venodilation, which reduces venous return to the heart. Decreased preload lowers myocardial oxygen demand. This relief of oxygen imbalance reduces anginal pain. It may also dilate coronary arteries to improve blood flow. The overall effect is decreased cardiac workload.

Q11. Answer: D

Explanation: Excessive chest tube drainage after cardiac surgery may indicate active bleeding. Rapid blood loss can lead to hypovolemia and hemodynamic instability. Immediate notification of the surgeon is required. Early intervention may prevent the need for reoperation. Continuous monitoring is essential in the postoperative period.

Q12. Answer: A

Explanation: Right-sided heart failure leads to systemic venous congestion. Fluid accumulates in dependent areas, causing peripheral edema. Jugular venous distension and hepatomegaly may also occur. Pulmonary symptoms are more typical of left-sided failure. Recognizing the distinction guides treatment strategies.

Q13. Answer: A

Explanation: Severe aortic stenosis obstructs blood flow from the left ventricle to the aorta. During exertion, cardiac output cannot increase adequately. This leads to decreased cerebral blood flow and syncope. The obstruction limits systemic perfusion under stress. Prompt evaluation is necessary to prevent sudden cardiac death.

Q14. Answer: B

Explanation: An INR of 5.5 indicates excessive anticoagulation. Holding the next dose reduces bleeding risk. Close monitoring is required to prevent hemorrhagic complications. Vitamin K may be considered if levels rise further or bleeding occurs. Proper dose adjustment ensures safe therapy.

Q15. Answer: B

Explanation: Sudden leg swelling and pain suggest deep vein thrombosis. Venous obstruction causes impaired return and localized inflammation. If untreated, embolization to the lungs may occur. Early anticoagulation reduces complications. Assessment and imaging confirm diagnosis.

Q16. Answer: A

Explanation: Ventricular fibrillation is a life-threatening arrhythmia characterized by chaotic electrical activity. Immediate defibrillation is required to restore organized rhythm. Early shock delivery significantly improves survival. Chest compressions are initiated if defibrillation is not immediately available. Rapid response is critical in cardiac arrest.

Q17. Answer: B

Explanation: Chronic venous insufficiency leads to prolonged venous hypertension. This causes hemosiderin deposition in the skin, producing brown discoloration. Edema and skin changes are common findings. Arterial disease presents differently with pale, cool limbs. Proper assessment distinguishes venous from arterial disorders.

Q18. Answer: B

Explanation: Pulmonary embolism obstructs pulmonary arterial flow. This results in sudden onset dyspnea and hypoxia. Chest pain and tachycardia may also occur. Prompt recognition and treatment are vital to prevent hemodynamic collapse. Early anticoagulation improves outcomes.

Q19. Answer: C

Explanation: Routine sedation interruption allows assessment for readiness to wean from ventilation. Reducing ventilation duration decreases pneumonia risk. Maintaining appropriate positioning and oral hygiene also contribute to prevention. Prolonged mechanical ventilation increases infection risk. Evidence-based bundles improve patient safety.

Q20. Answer: D

Explanation: Hypertensive crisis requires controlled reduction of blood pressure. Rapid excessive lowering can cause ischemia to vital organs. Gradual reduction minimizes risk of stroke or myocardial injury. Continuous monitoring is essential during treatment. Intravenous agents are often used for controlled response.

Q21. Answer: D

Explanation: Inferior wall myocardial infarction can extend to the right ventricle, impairing its pumping ability. Right ventricular dysfunction reduces blood flow to the left ventricle, leading to hypotension. Clear lung sounds indicate that pulmonary congestion is not present, which supports right-sided involvement. Reduced preload to the left heart further decreases cardiac output. Early recognition is essential because fluid administration may improve hemodynamics in this setting.

Q22. Answer: D

Explanation: Chronic hypertension increases afterload, forcing the left ventricle to work harder to eject blood. In response, myocardial fibers thicken to generate greater contractile force. This concentric hypertrophy initially maintains cardiac output. Over time, stiffened ventricular walls impair diastolic filling. Persistent pressure overload may eventually lead to heart failure.

Q23. Answer: A

Explanation: A 12-lead ECG is the fastest and most accessible diagnostic tool for suspected myocardial infarction. It identifies ST-segment changes and arrhythmias promptly. Early detection allows rapid initiation of reperfusion therapy. Time-sensitive management improves myocardial salvage. Additional imaging may follow but should not delay ECG acquisition.

Q24. Answer: C

Explanation: Hypoxia is suggested by low oxygen saturation and altered mental status. Immediate oxygen supplementation improves tissue oxygen delivery. Early correction prevents further deterioration. Ongoing monitoring determines the need for advanced airway support. Addressing hypoxia is the highest priority in this scenario.

Q25. Answer: A

Explanation: Mitral valve stenosis impedes blood flow from the left atrium to the left ventricle. Increased left atrial pressure backs up into pulmonary circulation. This leads to pulmonary congestion and dyspnea. Chronic pressure elevation may cause pulmonary hypertension. Early intervention prevents progressive heart failure.

Q26. Answer: D

Explanation: Reduced cardiac output decreases renal perfusion. The kidneys respond by lowering urine production. Oliguria is an early sign of impaired systemic perfusion. Continuous monitoring of intake and output helps detect deterioration. Prompt intervention may prevent renal injury.

Q27. Answer: D

Explanation: Pericarditis causes inflammation of the pericardial layers. Leaning forward reduces contact between inflamed surfaces. This decreases friction and alleviates pain. Pain is often sharp and worsens with inspiration or lying flat. Positional changes are characteristic in this condition.

Q28. Answer: B

Explanation: Digoxin toxicity commonly presents with gastrointestinal symptoms and visual disturbances. Elevated serum levels may cause arrhythmias and neurological changes. Renal dysfunction increases risk of accumulation. Monitoring serum levels and electrolytes is essential. Early identification prevents severe cardiac complications.

Q29. Answer: A

Explanation: Sequential compression devices promote venous return by applying intermittent pressure. This reduces venous stasis, a key factor in thrombosis formation. Early mobilization also supports prevention. Mechanical prophylaxis is especially important when anticoagulation is contraindicated. Preventive measures decrease risk of pulmonary embolism.

Q30. Answer: D

Explanation: ACE inhibitors block conversion of angiotensin I to angiotensin II. This reduces vasoconstriction and lowers systemic vascular resistance. Decreased afterload improves cardiac output. These agents also limit ventricular remodeling. Long-term use reduces morbidity and mortality in heart failure.

Q31. Answer: A

Explanation: Acute pulmonary edema causes fluid accumulation in alveoli. This results in frothy sputum that may appear pink due to capillary leakage. Crackles and severe dyspnea are common. Rapid intervention improves oxygenation. Untreated edema may lead to respiratory failure.

Q32. Answer: B

Explanation: Aortic dissection involves tearing of the aortic intima. Blood may obstruct branches supplying one arm, causing unequal pressures. Pain is often severe and tearing in nature. Immediate imaging and management are critical. Delay increases mortality risk.

Q33. Answer: D

Explanation: Hypokalemia affects cardiac repolarization. It may cause a prolonged QT interval and U waves. These changes increase risk of arrhythmias. Monitoring electrolytes prevents complications. Early correction stabilizes electrical activity.

Q34. Answer: D

Explanation: Ejection fraction measures the percentage of blood ejected during systole. A value of 25% indicates significant systolic impairment. Reduced contractility limits systemic perfusion. Patients are at high risk for heart failure symptoms. Guideline-directed therapy improves outcomes.

Q35. Answer: C

Explanation: Orthostatic hypotension occurs when blood pressure drops upon standing. Venous pooling reduces cerebral perfusion. Symptoms include dizziness and fainting. Gradual position changes help prevent episodes. Monitoring blood pressure in different positions aids diagnosis.

Q36. Answer: C

Explanation: Infective endocarditis causes vegetations on heart valves. Fragments may dislodge and travel to systemic circulation. Cerebral embolization can cause stroke. Early antibiotic therapy reduces risk. Ongoing monitoring detects complications promptly.

Q37. Answer: D

Explanation: Stable angina occurs due to predictable myocardial ischemia during exertion. Rest decreases oxygen demand and relieves symptoms. Episodes are typically brief and reproducible. Recognition distinguishes it from unstable angina. Proper management prevents progression.

Q38. Answer: C

Explanation: Atrial fibrillation leads to blood stasis in the atria. Clot formation increases risk of systemic embolization. Cerebral infarction is a serious complication. Anticoagulation significantly lowers this risk. Therapy must be carefully monitored.

Q39. Answer: B

Explanation: Severe anemia reduces oxygen-carrying capacity. The heart compensates by increasing cardiac output to deliver sufficient oxygen. This raises workload and may precipitate ischemia. Patients with coronary disease are particularly vulnerable. Correction improves oxygen delivery.

Q40. Answer: D

Explanation: Hypertrophic cardiomyopathy predisposes patients to malignant ventricular arrhythmias. Abnormal myocardial structure disrupts electrical conduction. Sudden cardiac death may occur without warning. Implantable defibrillators are often recommended for high-risk individuals. Early detection improves survival chances.

Q41. Answer: B

Explanation: Aspirin inhibits cyclooxygenase, which reduces thromboxane A2 production. This action decreases platelet aggregation and prevents further clot formation. Early administration limits thrombus growth in coronary arteries. It has been shown to reduce mortality in acute coronary syndromes. Prompt use is a standard evidence-based intervention.

Q42. Answer: B

Explanation: B-type natriuretic peptide is released in response to ventricular stretch and pressure overload. Elevated levels indicate increased cardiac wall tension. This biomarker assists in diagnosing and monitoring heart failure. Higher values often correlate with severity. Monitoring trends helps evaluate treatment effectiveness.

Q43. Answer: C

Explanation: Severe chest pain radiating to the back is classic for aortic dissection. A widened mediastinum on imaging further supports this diagnosis. The condition involves tearing of the aortic intima, allowing blood to track between layers. Rapid identification is critical due to high mortality. Immediate blood pressure control and surgical evaluation are essential.

Q44. Answer: A

Explanation: Second-degree type II block indicates intermittent failure of conduction from atria to ventricles. It often progresses to complete heart block. This can result in severe bradycardia and hemodynamic instability. Pacemaker insertion is frequently required. Continuous cardiac monitoring is essential for safety.

Q45. Answer: D

Explanation: Rest pain suggests severe arterial insufficiency. It indicates that blood flow is inadequate even without exertion. Nocturnal worsening occurs because gravity no longer assists perfusion. This stage carries a high risk for tissue loss. Urgent vascular evaluation is necessary.

Q46. Answer: A

Explanation: Rapid removal of pericardial fluid can lead to sudden changes in cardiac filling dynamics. The abrupt increase in venous return may cause reflex vasodilation. This can result in transient hypotension. Gradual drainage helps minimize hemodynamic instability. Close monitoring is required during the procedure.

Q47. Answer: A

Explanation: Atrial flutter commonly produces atrial rates around 300 beats per minute. A 2:1 conduction pattern often results in a ventricular rate of 150. The characteristic sawtooth pattern appears on ECG. Rate control and rhythm management are primary goals. Untreated rapid rates may cause cardiomyopathy.

Q48. Answer: B

Explanation: Furosemide is a loop diuretic that promotes sodium and water excretion. This reduces circulating blood volume. Lower volume decreases venous return to the heart. Reduced preload alleviates pulmonary congestion. Monitoring electrolytes is important during therapy.

Q49. Answer: B

Explanation: Exercise-induced chest pain relieved by rest is typical of stable angina. It results from transient imbalance between oxygen supply and demand. Fixed atherosclerotic narrowing limits blood flow during exertion. Rest reduces myocardial workload. The condition requires risk factor management.

Q50. Answer: B

Explanation: Calcium gluconate stabilizes the myocardial cell membrane. It reduces the risk of life-threatening arrhythmias. This intervention acts rapidly but does not lower potassium levels. Additional therapies shift potassium intracellularly or remove it. Continuous ECG monitoring is necessary.

Q51. Answer: A

Explanation: Vegetations from infected heart valves can embolize to systemic organs. Renal embolization may cause flank pain and hematuria. This represents a serious complication. Prompt imaging and antibiotic therapy are critical. Early treatment limits organ damage.

Q52. Answer: C

Explanation: An S3 sound occurs during early diastole when blood rapidly fills a dilated ventricle. It is often associated with volume overload. In adults, it commonly indicates heart failure. The sound reflects decreased ventricular compliance. Recognition aids clinical assessment.

Q53. Answer: B

Explanation: Mechanical valves are prone to clot formation due to artificial surfaces. Thrombi may embolize and cause stroke. Long-term anticoagulation reduces this risk. Careful monitoring ensures therapeutic levels. Patient education improves adherence and safety.

Q54. Answer: B

Explanation: Prolonged immobility increases risk of deep vein thrombosis. A clot may travel to the pulmonary arteries. Sudden dyspnea is a hallmark symptom. Early anticoagulation reduces morbidity. Rapid evaluation is essential to prevent deterioration.

Q55. Answer: D

Explanation: Inotropic agents enhance myocardial contractility. Improved contractile strength increases cardiac output. This helps restore tissue perfusion. Close monitoring prevents arrhythmias. The therapy supports failing myocardium during acute episodes.

Q56. Answer: B

Explanation: Sodium promotes water retention in the body. Excess volume increases blood pressure. Reducing sodium lowers circulating fluid volume. This helps decrease vascular resistance. Lifestyle modifications are essential components of hypertension management.

Q57. Answer: C

Explanation: Narrow QRS complexes indicate that ventricular conduction is intact. A rapid regular rhythm suggests supraventricular tachycardia. Symptoms result from reduced ventricular filling time. Vagal maneuvers or medications may terminate the episode. Persistent cases require further intervention.

Q58. Answer: C

Explanation: Impaired renal function reduces potassium excretion. Elevated potassium levels affect cardiac conduction. Severe hyperkalemia may cause arrhythmias. Monitoring serum electrolytes is critical in renal patients. Early treatment prevents life-threatening events.

Q59. Answer: D

Explanation: Papillary muscles anchor mitral valve leaflets. Ischemic damage may impair their function. This leads to improper valve closure during systole. Acute mitral regurgitation can cause pulmonary edema. Rapid recognition is vital for management.

Q60. Answer: C

Explanation: Elevated lactate levels indicate anaerobic metabolism. This occurs when tissues do not receive adequate oxygen. High lactate is a marker of poor perfusion. Serial measurements assess response to therapy. Early correction improves survival outcomes.

Q61. Answer: A

Explanation: ST elevation in inferior leads with hypotension and clear lungs suggests right ventricular involvement. Right ventricular infarction reduces preload to the left ventricle. Fluid administration helps improve ventricular filling and cardiac output. Vasodilators could worsen hypotension in this setting. Early hemodynamic stabilization improves survival.

Q62. Answer: B

Explanation: Minimal chest tube drainage with acute dyspnea may indicate clot obstruction and fluid accumulation. Tamponade compresses the heart and limits filling. Tachycardia occurs as compensation for reduced stroke volume. Oxygen saturation decreases due to poor perfusion. Immediate evaluation with echocardiography is essential.

Q63. Answer: D

Explanation: Omission of diuretics leads to fluid accumulation. Signs of decompensation include edema and orthopnea. Prompt diuretic administration reduces volume overload. Improved fluid balance decreases pulmonary congestion. Early treatment prevents further deterioration.

Q64. Answer: D

Explanation: A very high INR increases risk of bleeding. Severe headache raises concern for intracranial hemorrhage. Vitamin K reverses excessive anticoagulation. Immediate correction reduces risk of fatal bleeding. Close neurological monitoring is required.

Q65. Answer: A

Explanation: Persistent hypotension with high filling pressures indicates pump failure. Low cardiac output despite adequate volume suggests myocardial dysfunction. Sepsis can depress cardiac contractility. Elevated preload with poor output characterizes cardiogenic shock. Early inotropic support may be necessary.

Q66. Answer: C

Explanation: Hypertrophic cardiomyopathy predisposes patients to lethal ventricular arrhythmias. Sudden collapse during exertion suggests arrhythmic event. An implantable defibrillator detects and terminates dangerous rhythms. This significantly reduces sudden cardiac death risk. Preventive device therapy is recommended in high-risk patients.

Q67. Answer: C

Explanation: Severe aortic stenosis limits cardiac output and causes exertional symptoms. Syncope and angina indicate advanced disease. Valve replacement restores forward blood flow. Medical therapy alone does not correct mechanical obstruction. Early surgical evaluation improves prognosis.

Q68. Answer: A

Explanation: Amiodarone can depress myocardial conduction and contractility. Bradycardia with hypotension suggests adverse drug effect. Temporary discontinuation allows hemodynamic stabilization. Continuous monitoring ensures patient safety. Dose adjustment may be required before restarting therapy.

Q69. Answer: A

Explanation: Presentation suggests acute aortic dissection. High blood pressure increases shear stress on the aorta. Rapid controlled reduction decreases further tearing. Thrombolytics are contraindicated. Early stabilization reduces mortality risk.

Q70. Answer: B

Explanation: Chronic atrial fibrillation promotes clot formation in atria. Embolization to cerebral circulation causes ischemic stroke. Sudden neurological deficits confirm acute event. Immediate evaluation for reperfusion therapy is required. Preventive anticoagulation reduces this risk.

Q71. Answer: C

Explanation: A new systolic murmur after infarction suggests structural damage. Septal rupture allows abnormal blood flow between ventricles. This leads to acute volume overload and pulmonary edema. It is a life-threatening complication. Immediate surgical consultation is required.

Q72. Answer: B

Explanation: Massive pulmonary embolism with hypotension indicates hemodynamic instability. Thrombolytics rapidly dissolve clot burden. Restoring pulmonary circulation improves cardiac output. Delayed treatment increases mortality. Immediate intervention is critical.

Q73. Answer: B

Explanation: Hypokalemia increases myocardial excitability. This predisposes to dangerous ventricular arrhythmias. Diuretic therapy commonly lowers potassium levels. Prompt correction stabilizes cardiac conduction. Continuous monitoring prevents sudden deterioration.

Q74. Answer: A

Explanation: Troponin may not elevate immediately after myocardial injury. Serial measurements detect rising levels. Early discharge could miss evolving infarction. Ongoing monitoring ensures accurate diagnosis. Time-based testing improves detection.

Q75. Answer: B

Explanation: Mitral regurgitation allows blood to flow backward into the left atrium. This increases atrial volume and pressure. Pulmonary congestion may result. Over time, ventricular dilation occurs. Progressive symptoms require evaluation for surgical repair.

Q76. Answer: B

Explanation: Certain patients with valvular disease require antibiotic prophylaxis. Dental procedures may introduce bacteria into bloodstream. Preventing bacteremia reduces endocarditis risk. Evidence-based guidelines support this approach. Proper timing ensures effectiveness.

Q77. Answer: C

Explanation: Unstable ventricular tachycardia requires immediate intervention. Hypotension and altered mental status indicate poor perfusion. Synchronized cardioversion restores organized rhythm. Delay may lead to cardiac arrest. Rapid action improves survival.

Q78. Answer: C

Explanation: Venous ulcers result from chronic venous hypertension. Compression improves venous return and reduces edema. Proper wound care supports healing. Early treatment prevents progression. Patient education enhances compliance.

Q79. Answer: D

Explanation: Inferior myocardial infarction may involve the vagus nerve. Increased parasympathetic tone slows heart rate. Bradycardia can reduce cardiac output and cause hypotension. Atropine may be required. Close monitoring ensures timely intervention.

Q80. Answer: C

Explanation: High sodium intake promotes water retention. Increased volume elevates preload and pulmonary pressures. Fluid accumulation in lungs causes dyspnea and crackles. Managing dietary intake prevents exacerbations. Patient education is essential for long-term control.

Q81. Answer: B

Explanation: This presentation is consistent with hypertensive emergency due to end-organ damage. Papilledema indicates increased intracranial pressure. Blood pressure must be reduced in a controlled and gradual manner using intravenous agents. Rapid excessive reduction can compromise cerebral perfusion. Careful monitoring in a critical care setting is required.

Q82. Answer: C

Explanation: Anterior wall infarctions commonly affect the left ventricle. Impaired contractility leads to decreased cardiac output and pulmonary congestion. Bilateral crackles indicate fluid accumulation in alveoli. Hypotension reflects reduced systemic perfusion. Immediate supportive therapy is necessary to stabilize the patient.

Q83. Answer: B

Explanation: Bleeding is a serious complication of thrombolytic therapy. Oozing from IV sites suggests systemic fibrinolysis. The infusion should be stopped immediately to prevent further hemorrhage. Rapid assessment and provider notification are essential. Early intervention reduces risk of major bleeding events.

Q84. Answer: B

Explanation: ACE inhibitors reduce afterload and prevent ventricular remodeling. They improve symptoms and decrease mortality in systolic heart failure. Lowering systemic resistance enhances forward blood flow. Long-term therapy slows disease progression. Evidence supports their routine use in reduced ejection fraction.

Q85. Answer: A

Explanation: Central line placement can cause lung puncture. Air accumulation in the pleural space compresses the lung and mediastinum. Hypotension results from impaired venous return. Absent breath sounds on one side are characteristic. Immediate needle decompression is required.

Q86. Answer: A

Explanation: Rapid ventricular response with hemodynamic instability requires urgent cardioversion. Hypotension indicates poor perfusion. Electrical cardioversion restores organized rhythm quickly. Delayed treatment increases risk of shock. Stabilization is the immediate priority.

Q87. Answer: A

Explanation: Peripheral arterial disease reduces blood supply to distal tissues. Poor oxygen delivery impairs wound healing. Pale skin indicates diminished perfusion. Chronic ischemia increases risk of tissue necrosis. Vascular evaluation is essential for management.

Q88. Answer: A

Explanation: Spironolactone conserves potassium while promoting sodium excretion. Excess potassium accumulation can occur, especially with renal impairment. Elevated levels may cause muscle weakness and arrhythmias. Monitoring serum potassium is crucial. Dose adjustment may be required to prevent complications.

Q89. Answer: C

Explanation: A bruit at the insertion site suggests turbulent blood flow. Pseudoaneurysm forms when blood leaks into surrounding tissue but remains connected to artery. Swelling and pulsation are typical findings. Ultrasound confirms diagnosis. Early intervention prevents rupture.

Q90. Answer: B

Explanation: Vegetations on heart valves may fragment and embolize. Cerebral arteries are common targets. Sudden neurological deficit indicates possible stroke. Rapid neuroimaging is necessary. Early treatment improves neurological outcomes.

Q91. Answer: B

Explanation: Improved urine output reflects better renal perfusion. It is an early sign of improved cardiac output. Monitoring hourly output guides therapy. Decreasing lactate would also indicate improvement, but urine output is a direct bedside measure. Adequate perfusion is the treatment goal.

Q92. Answer: C

Explanation: Unstable angina presents with rest pain without biomarker elevation. It indicates high risk for progression to infarction. Early dual antiplatelet and anticoagulation therapy prevents clot extension. Close monitoring is required. Aggressive management reduces adverse outcomes.

Q93. Answer: A

Explanation: Anemia lowers hemoglobin concentration. Reduced oxygen transport leads to myocardial ischemia. Patients with coronary disease are especially vulnerable. The heart compensates by increasing workload. Correcting anemia improves oxygen delivery.

Q94. Answer: B

Explanation: Chronic hypertension damages renal vasculature. Narrowed arteries reduce blood flow to nephrons. Sustained injury impairs filtration. Progressive scarring leads to chronic kidney disease. Blood pressure control slows progression.

Q95. Answer: A

Explanation: Pink frothy sputum indicates acute pulmonary edema. Oxygen improves gas exchange. Diuretics reduce fluid overload. Upright positioning also aids breathing. Rapid treatment prevents respiratory failure.

Q96. Answer: B

Explanation: Atrial fibrillation longer than 48 hours increases thrombus risk. Cardioversion may dislodge clot. Adequate anticoagulation reduces embolic risk. Transesophageal echocardiography may also be performed. Proper preparation prevents stroke.

Q97. Answer: A

Explanation: Early septic shock causes vasodilation. Warm skin and bounding pulses result from increased cardiac output. Hypotension may still be present. Later stages show cool extremities. Early recognition allows timely intervention.

Q98. Answer: D

Explanation: Pulmonary hypertension increases resistance in pulmonary arteries. The right ventricle must pump against higher pressure. Chronic strain leads to right ventricular hypertrophy and failure. Edema results from systemic congestion. Early treatment targets pulmonary pressures.

Q99. Answer: A

Explanation: Recurrent ST elevation after angioplasty suggests vessel re-occlusion. Acute thrombosis can occur at stent site. Immediate evaluation is required. Delay may lead to myocardial damage. Rapid reperfusion improves outcomes.

Q100. Answer: A

Explanation: Severe hypotension with signs of poor perfusion indicates cardiogenic shock. Cool extremities and confusion reflect decreased cerebral and systemic blood flow. Cardiac output is critically reduced. Immediate hemodynamic support is necessary. Early intervention improves survival rates.

Question (101-200)

Q101. Which principle best explains why increased afterload reduces stroke volume in systolic heart failure?

(A) Increased resistance to ventricular ejection
(B) Decreased ventricular filling time
(C) Enhanced venous return
(D) Reduced myocardial oxygen extraction

Q102. Why does chronic mitral stenosis commonly lead to atrial fibrillation?

(A) Reduced pulmonary vascular resistance
(B) Decreased ventricular compliance
(C) Increased right ventricular contractility
(D) Left atrial enlargement from pressure overload

Q103. What is the conceptual reason beta-blockers reduce mortality after myocardial infarction?

(A) They decrease myocardial oxygen demand
(B) They increase heart rate
(C) They increase preload
(D) They promote platelet aggregation

Q104. Why does right-sided heart failure cause peripheral edema?

(A) Decreased sodium excretion alone
(B) Increased pulmonary capillary pressure
(C) Elevated systemic venous pressure
(D) Reduced left ventricular output only

Q105. What is the underlying concept behind using diuretics in acute pulmonary edema?

(A) Increase myocardial contractility
(B) Stimulate respiratory center
(C) Decrease intravascular volume and preload
(D) Improve coronary artery dilation

Q106. Why is troponin considered more specific than CK-MB for myocardial injury?

(A) It rises earlier than CK-MB
(B) It remains elevated for weeks only
(C) It is found in skeletal muscle predominantly
(D) It is unique to cardiac muscle tissue

Q107. What is the physiologic basis for orthopnea in heart failure?

(A) Redistribution of fluid to lungs when supine
(B) Decreased heart rate at night
(C) Increased hemoglobin concentration
(D) Reduced renal perfusion

Q108. Why does hyperkalemia increase the risk of cardiac arrhythmias?

(A) It reduces atrial size
(B) It increases hemoglobin binding
(C) It alters resting membrane potential
(D) It decreases myocardial excitability

Q109. What is the main reason anticoagulation is required in atrial fibrillation?

(A) Lower systemic blood pressure
(B) Prevent ventricular hypertrophy
(C) Increase cardiac output
(D) Reduce blood stasis in atria

Q110. Why does aortic stenosis lead to concentric left ventricular hypertrophy?

(A) Reduced stroke volume
(B) Increased preload
(C) Increased afterload
(D) Decreased coronary flow

Q111. What explains the development of an S3 heart sound in systolic heart failure?

(A) Atrial contraction against stiff ventricle
(B) Pericardial inflammation
(C) Rapid filling of a dilated ventricle
(D) Valve calcification

Q112. Why are ACE inhibitors beneficial in preventing ventricular remodeling after myocardial infarction?

(A) They increase aldosterone secretion
(B) They block angiotensin II effects
(C) They enhance platelet function
(D) They raise systemic vascular resistance

Q113. What is the physiologic reason hypotension occurs in cardiac tamponade?

(A) Impaired ventricular filling
(B) Elevated hemoglobin levels
(C) Excess systemic vasodilation
(D) Increased myocardial contractility

Q114. Why is gradual blood pressure reduction recommended in hypertensive emergency?

(A) To increase renal output rapidly
(B) To prevent reflex tachycardia
(C) To maintain organ perfusion
(D) To stimulate sympathetic tone

Q115. What is the conceptual basis for using compression stockings in venous insufficiency?

(A) Increase arterial blood flow
(B) Decrease heart rate
(C) Stimulate lymph production

(D) Reduce venous pooling

Q116. Why does severe anemia increase cardiac workload?

(A) It increases systemic resistance
(B) It reduces oxygen-carrying capacity
(C) It decreases stroke volume
(D) It raises blood viscosity

Q117. What explains the mechanism of action of nitrates in angina management?

(A) Dilate veins reducing preload
(B) Promote clot formation
(C) Stimulate sympathetic response
(D) Increase heart rate

Q118. Why does pulmonary embolism cause sudden dyspnea?

(A) Enhanced oxygen diffusion
(B) Obstruction of pulmonary blood flow
(C) Increased left ventricular output
(D) Reduced respiratory drive

Q119. What is the rationale behind using statins in coronary artery disease?

(A) Raise blood pressure
(B) Increase triglyceride absorption
(C) Increase platelet adhesion
(D) Lower LDL cholesterol and stabilize plaques

Q120. Why does left ventricular failure often lead to pulmonary hypertension?

(A) Backward transmission of elevated left atrial pressure
(B) Reduced hemoglobin levels
(C) Decreased venous return
(D) Increased systemic resistance

Q121. A 62-year-old male with history of smoking presents to the emergency department with sudden onset chest pain and shortness of breath. ECG shows ST elevation in leads V1-V4. Blood pressure is 100/60 mmHg and crackles are heard bilaterally. What is the most likely complication developing?

(A) Atrial septal defect
(B) Acute left ventricular failure
(C) Pericarditis
(D) Right ventricular infarction

Q122. A 70-year-old female with chronic atrial fibrillation stops taking anticoagulation medication. Two days later she develops sudden right arm weakness and difficulty speaking. What is the underlying mechanism?

(A) Embolic stroke from atrial thrombus
(B) Intracranial tumor
(C) Hypoglycemia
(D) Cerebral vasospasm

Q123. A patient one hour after cardiac catheterization develops swelling, pain, and a pulsatile mass at the femoral site. What complication should be suspected?

(A) Pseudoaneurysm
(B) Deep vein thrombosis
(C) Cellulitis
(D) Hemothorax

Q124. A 55-year-old man with uncontrolled hypertension presents with tearing chest pain radiating to his back. Blood pressure differs by 30 mmHg between arms. What is the most appropriate immediate management?

(A) Provide oral nitrates only
(B) Encourage ambulation
(C) Administer IV beta-blocker to lower blood pressure
(D) Start thrombolytic therapy

Q125. A patient with heart failure presents with increasing shortness of breath when lying flat and requires three pillows at night. What is the pathophysiologic explanation?

(A) Fluid redistribution to pulmonary circulation
(B) Decreased hemoglobin
(C) Increased renal perfusion
(D) Reduced systemic resistance

Q126. A patient with infective endocarditis develops sudden flank pain and hematuria. What is the most likely cause?

(A) Dehydration
(B) Renal embolism
(C) Urinary tract infection
(D) Kidney stone

Q127. A 68-year-old patient with severe aortic stenosis experiences syncope while climbing stairs. What is the primary reason for syncope?

(A) Hypoglycemia
(B) Hyperkalemia
(C) Decreased cerebral perfusion during exertion
(D) Increased venous return

Q128. A patient with acute pulmonary embolism becomes hypotensive and confused. What is occurring physiologically?

(A) Decreased systemic vascular resistance only
(B) Hypervolemia
(C) Obstruction of pulmonary circulation reducing cardiac output
(D) Increased left ventricular preload

Q129. A patient receiving digoxin presents with nausea, blurred vision, and irregular pulse. What factor increases risk of this toxicity?
(A) Hyperkalemia
(B) Elevated hemoglobin
(C) Hypokalemia
(D) Hypernatremia

Q130. A 60-year-old diabetic patient develops a non-healing ulcer on the lateral toe with diminished pedal pulses. What is the underlying problem?
(A) Allergic dermatitis
(B) Lymphatic obstruction
(C) Arterial insufficiency
(D) Venous insufficiency

Q131. A patient post-myocardial infarction suddenly develops severe dyspnea and a new loud systolic murmur. What mechanical complication is most likely?
(A) Papillary muscle rupture
(B) First-degree AV block
(C) Pericarditis
(D) Sinus tachycardia

Q132. A patient with cardiogenic shock has cool extremities and decreased urine output despite adequate fluid resuscitation. What medication is most appropriate?
(A) Inotropic agent
(B) Sedative
(C) Antacid
(D) Antibiotic

Q133. A patient develops bradycardia and hypotension after inferior myocardial infarction. What is the likely cause?
(A) Dehydration
(B) Increased vagal tone
(C) Sympathetic overactivity
(D) Hyperthyroidism

Q134. A patient with long-standing hypertension presents with left ventricular hypertrophy on echocardiogram. What is the compensatory mechanism?
(A) Valve insufficiency
(B) Volume overload adaptation
(C) Reduced contractility
(D) Pressure overload adaptation

Q135. A patient with chronic heart failure gains 4 pounds in three days and has ankle swelling. What should the nurse advise?
(A) Take extra diuretic as prescribed
(B) Limit rest
(C) Stop all medications
(D) Increase sodium intake

Q136. A patient experiences sudden collapse and ECG shows chaotic irregular waveform without identifiable QRS complexes. What rhythm is present?
(A) Sinus rhythm
(B) Ventricular fibrillation
(C) First-degree block
(D) Atrial flutter

Q137. A patient with severe anemia and coronary artery disease reports chest discomfort during minimal activity. What is the cause?
(A) Reduced oxygen delivery to myocardium
(B) Increased preload
(C) Decreased afterload
(D) Increased oxygen supply

Q138. A patient with pulmonary hypertension develops bilateral lower extremity edema and hepatomegaly. What cardiac chamber is primarily affected?
(A) Right ventricle
(B) Aorta
(C) Left atrium
(D) Left ventricle

Q139. A patient with unstable angina continues to have chest pain at rest despite medication. What is the next step?
(A) Discharge home
(B) Urgent coronary angiography
(C) Recommend exercise
(D) Prescribe antibiotics

Q140. A patient develops confusion, hypotension, and cool clammy skin after large myocardial infarction. What condition is occurring?
(A) Stable angina
(B) Controlled hypertension

(C) Cardiogenic shock
(D) Hyperthyroidism

Q141. A 65-year-old male with history of myocardial infarction presents with progressive shortness of breath and swelling of both legs. On examination, jugular venous distension and hepatomegaly are noted. What is the most likely pathophysiologic process?
(A) Acute pulmonary embolism
(B) Right-sided heart failure secondary to left failure
(C) Left ventricular hypertrophy
(D) Mitral valve prolapse

Q142. A patient undergoing hemodialysis complains of chest pain and hypotension shortly after the session begins. ECG shows peaked T waves. What is the most likely electrolyte imbalance?
(A) Hyponatremia
(B) Hypocalcemia
(C) Hypokalemia
(D) Hyperkalemia

Q143. A 72-year-old woman with atrial fibrillation presents with sudden severe abdominal pain and absent bowel sounds. What complication should be suspected?
(A) Constipation
(B) Gastritis
(C) Appendicitis
(D) Mesenteric ischemia from embolism

Q144. A patient one week after myocardial infarction develops sharp chest pain that worsens with inspiration and improves when leaning forward. What condition is most likely?
(A) Aortic stenosis
(B) Pericarditis
(C) Pulmonary edema
(D) Reinfarction

Q145. A patient with chronic hypertension suddenly develops weakness on one side and difficulty speaking. CT scan shows intracerebral hemorrhage. What is the primary cause?
(A) Infection
(B) Vessel rupture due to long-standing high pressure
(C) Embolic event
(D) Hypoglycemia

Q146. A 59-year-old patient with stable angina reports chest discomfort when climbing stairs that resolves within minutes of rest. What does this indicate about coronary blood flow?
(A) Complete occlusion at rest
(B) Increased myocardial oxygen supply
(C) Excessive coronary dilation
(D) Adequate flow at rest but insufficient during exertion

Q147. A patient receiving intravenous fluids rapidly for septic shock develops increasing crackles and hypoxia. What complication is developing?
(A) Stroke
(B) Pericarditis
(C) Renal infarction
(D) Cardiogenic pulmonary edema

Q148. A patient with severe mitral regurgitation develops atrial fibrillation. What structural change most likely contributed?
(A) Right ventricular hypertrophy
(B) Left atrial dilation
(C) Aortic narrowing
(D) Pulmonary valve stenosis

Q149. A patient collapses and is found pulseless with ventricular tachycardia on monitor. What is the immediate action?
(A) Synchronized cardioversion
(B) Oxygen by nasal cannula
(C) Oral medication
(D) Defibrillation

Q150. A patient with advanced heart failure reports decreased urine output and confusion. Blood pressure is 82/48 mmHg. What stage is likely present?
(A) Controlled hypertension
(B) Stable angina
(C) Cardiogenic shock
(D) Compensated heart failure

Q151. A patient with infective endocarditis develops small, painless hemorrhagic lesions on palms and soles. What are these lesions indicative of?
(A) Septic emboli
(B) Fungal infection
(C) Allergic reaction
(D) Hyperlipidemia

Q152. A 67-year-old with peripheral arterial disease complains of calf pain after walking one block that resolves with rest. What physiologic process causes this pain?
(A) Venous congestion
(B) Lymphatic obstruction
(C) Muscle strain
(D) Ischemia due to increased oxygen demand
Q153. A patient with chronic kidney disease presents with chest pain and pericardial friction rub. What is the likely diagnosis?
(A) Pulmonary embolism
(B) Myocardial infarction
(C) Stable angina
(D) Uremic pericarditis
Q154. A patient after valve replacement surgery develops fever and positive blood cultures. What complication should be suspected?
(A) Valve thrombosis
(B) Hypokalemia
(C) Heart block
(D) Prosthetic valve endocarditis
Q155. A patient with pulmonary embolism reports pleuritic chest pain and hemoptysis. What is the pathophysiologic explanation?
(A) Pulmonary infarction
(B) Hypervolemia
(C) Reduced oxygen consumption
(D) Increased left ventricular pressure
Q156. A 74-year-old patient with uncontrolled diabetes develops silent myocardial infarction. Why might chest pain be absent?
(A) Hyperkalemia
(B) Valve stenosis
(C) Autonomic neuropathy
(D) Increased sympathetic tone
Q157. A patient with severe heart failure develops Cheyne-Stokes respirations during sleep. What is the cause?
(A) Delayed circulation time affecting respiratory control
(B) Infection
(C) Airway obstruction
(D) Increased respiratory drive
Q158. A patient with deep vein thrombosis suddenly becomes hypotensive and tachycardic. What is the most serious concern?
(A) Stroke
(B) Pulmonary embolism
(C) Pericardial effusion
(D) Myocarditis
Q159. A patient with cardiomyopathy develops sustained ventricular tachycardia. What is the underlying substrate for this arrhythmia?
(A) Decreased sympathetic tone
(B) Enhanced oxygen delivery
(C) Myocardial scar and electrical instability
(D) Valve calcification
Q160. A patient presents with sudden onset severe dyspnea, hypotension, distended neck veins, and clear lung sounds after chest trauma. What condition is most likely?
(A) Acute asthma
(B) Pulmonary edema
(C) Pneumonia
(D) Cardiac tamponade
Q161. A 63-year-old patient with history of coronary artery disease presents with sudden onset chest pain at rest lasting 30 minutes. ECG shows ST depression in multiple leads. Troponin is mildly elevated. What is the most likely diagnosis?
(A) NSTEMI
(B) Pericarditis
(C) Stable angina
(D) Aortic dissection
Q162. A patient with severe heart failure is started on high-dose diuretics and later develops dizziness and hypotension. What is the likely mechanism?
(A) Elevated systemic resistance
(B) Increased preload
(C) Excessive volume depletion
(D) Hyperkalemia
Q163. A patient presents with sudden tearing chest pain and syncope. Imaging confirms ascending aortic dissection. What is the definitive treatment?
(A) Emergency surgical repair
(B) Oral antihypertensives only
(C) Bed rest alone
(D) Thrombolytic therapy
Q164. A patient with chronic atrial fibrillation reports increasing fatigue and shortness of

breath. Heart rate is persistently 140 bpm. What complication is developing?
(A) Pulmonary embolism
(B) Pericardial effusion
(C) Tachycardia-induced cardiomyopathy
(D) Valve stenosis

Q165. A patient post-myocardial infarction develops hypotension and a new harsh holosystolic murmur. What structural defect is most likely?
(A) Aortic regurgitation
(B) Ventricular septal rupture
(C) Pulmonary stenosis
(D) Tricuspid prolapse

Q166. A patient with deep vein thrombosis is started on anticoagulation. Two days later, sudden chest pain and dyspnea occur. What is the likely explanation?
(A) Hyperventilation syndrome
(B) Pulmonary embolism
(C) Drug allergy
(D) Myocardial infarction

Q167. A patient with hypertrophic cardiomyopathy experiences worsening symptoms after taking a vasodilator. Why might this occur?
(A) Reduced heart rate
(B) Increased afterload
(C) Decreased preload worsening obstruction
(D) Enhanced myocardial perfusion

Q168. A patient presents with hypotension, muffled heart sounds, and distended neck veins after chest trauma. What immediate procedure is required?
(A) Intravenous antibiotics
(B) Intubation
(C) Chest physiotherapy
(D) Pericardiocentesis

Q169. A patient with severe anemia and tachycardia develops signs of heart failure. What is the primary trigger?
(A) Elevated platelet count
(B) Decreased systemic resistance
(C) Increased blood viscosity
(D) Reduced oxygen delivery causing compensatory overload

Q170. A patient with end-stage renal disease develops pericardial effusion. What is the underlying cause?
(A) Coronary plaque rupture
(B) Hyperlipidemia
(C) Bacterial infection
(D) Uremic toxin accumulation

Q171. A patient with pulmonary embolism has elevated jugular venous pressure and clear lungs. What is the reason for neck vein distension?
(A) Right ventricular strain
(B) Hypervolemia
(C) Left ventricular failure
(D) Mitral stenosis

Q172. A patient with uncontrolled hypertension develops concentric left ventricular hypertrophy. Over time, what complication may result?
(A) Reduced myocardial stiffness
(B) Diastolic dysfunction
(C) Hyperdynamic circulation
(D) Improved systolic function

Q173. A patient develops sudden dyspnea and hypotension during hemodialysis. Breath sounds are diminished on one side. What complication is suspected?
(A) Myocardial infarction
(B) Pneumothorax
(C) Pulmonary edema
(D) Stroke

Q174. A patient with advanced heart failure reports paroxysmal nocturnal dyspnea. What causes this symptom?
(A) Decreased renal perfusion
(B) Fluid reabsorption into circulation during sleep
(C) Decreased systemic resistance
(D) Increased hemoglobin

Q175. A patient with infective endocarditis develops splinter hemorrhages under fingernails. What is the underlying cause?
(A) Vitamin deficiency
(B) Microemboli from valve vegetations
(C) Fungal infection
(D) Platelet deficiency

Q176. A patient collapses and monitor shows asystole. What is the immediate management?

(A) Oral medication
(B) High-quality CPR and epinephrine
(C) Defibrillation
(D) Synchronized cardioversion

Q177. A patient with severe mitral stenosis develops hemoptysis. What explains this symptom?
(A) Increased systemic pressure
(B) Aortic rupture
(C) Dehydration
(D) Pulmonary venous hypertension

Q178. A patient with dilated cardiomyopathy experiences worsening fatigue and hypotension. Echocardiogram shows EF 20%. What device may improve survival?
(A) Pacemaker for bradycardia only
(B) Temporary oxygen therapy
(C) Oral antacid
(D) Implantable cardioverter-defibrillator

Q179. A patient with acute myocardial infarction develops nausea, bradycardia, and hypotension. Which infarct location is most likely?
(A) Septal wall
(B) Lateral wall
(C) Anterior wall
(D) Inferior wall

Q180. A patient with severe heart failure presents with lactic acidosis and cool extremities. What is the primary cause of lactic acidosis?
(A) Anaerobic metabolism from poor perfusion
(B) Hyperventilation
(C) Increased oxygen delivery
(D) Excess sodium intake

Q181. A 69-year-old male with history of heart failure presents with increasing shortness of breath, pink frothy sputum, and severe anxiety. Blood pressure is 170/100 mmHg. What is the immediate priority treatment?
(A) Lay patient flat
(B) Delay intervention for imaging
(C) Administer high-flow oxygen and IV diuretic
(D) Encourage oral fluids

Q182. A patient with chronic atrial fibrillation is scheduled for elective hip surgery. What is the primary concern when stopping anticoagulation preoperatively?
(A) Increased risk of thromboembolism
(B) Hyperkalemia
(C) Hypoglycemia
(D) Hypertension

Q183. A 58-year-old woman with severe aortic regurgitation complains of bounding pulses and head bobbing. What is the underlying hemodynamic change?
(A) Increased systemic resistance
(B) Wide pulse pressure
(C) Decreased stroke volume
(D) Reduced preload

Q184. A patient with acute myocardial infarction suddenly becomes confused and hypotensive. Urine output drops significantly. What complication is most likely?
(A) Stable angina
(B) Hyperthyroidism
(C) Pericarditis
(D) Cardiogenic shock

Q185. A patient presents with chest pain and ECG shows diffuse ST elevation with PR depression. Troponin levels are normal. What is the most likely diagnosis?
(A) NSTEMI
(B) Pericarditis
(C) STEMI
(D) Pulmonary embolism

Q186. A patient with dilated cardiomyopathy develops worsening lower extremity edema and ascites. What mechanism explains fluid accumulation?
(A) Increased systemic venous congestion
(B) Reduced venous pressure
(C) Decreased aldosterone activity
(D) Increased oncotic pressure

Q187. A patient with pulmonary embolism is started on anticoagulation. What is the main therapeutic goal?
(A) Lower blood glucose
(B) Increase heart rate
(C) Prevent further clot propagation
(D) Dissolve clot immediately in all cases

Q188. A 66-year-old patient with long-standing hypertension develops exertional dyspnea. Echocardiogram shows preserved ejection fraction but thickened ventricular walls. What type of heart failure is present?

(A) Diastolic heart failure
(B) High-output failure
(C) Systolic heart failure
(D) Right-sided failure only

Q189. A patient receiving thrombolytics for acute myocardial infarction develops sudden severe headache and vomiting. What is the immediate concern?
(A) Hyperglycemia
(B) Anxiety
(C) Intracranial hemorrhage
(D) Migraine

Q190. A patient with peripheral arterial disease reports numbness and pale, cool toes. Capillary refill is delayed. What stage is likely present?
(A) Critical limb ischemia
(B) Hypervolemia
(C) Lymphatic obstruction
(D) Mild venous congestion

Q191. A patient with infective endocarditis develops acute shortness of breath and hypotension. Echocardiogram reveals severe valve destruction. What is the likely outcome if untreated?
(A) Acute heart failure
(B) Hypoglycemia
(C) Hyperlipidemia
(D) Spontaneous recovery

Q192. A patient with chronic heart failure experiences sudden palpitations and dizziness. ECG shows wide complex tachycardia. What is the most concerning rhythm?
(A) First-degree block
(B) Atrial flutter
(C) Ventricular tachycardia
(D) Sinus tachycardia

Q193. A patient with mitral stenosis presents with hemoptysis and dyspnea. What pathophysiologic change causes these symptoms?
(A) Increased cardiac output
(B) Reduced right atrial pressure
(C) Decreased systemic resistance
(D) Pulmonary venous congestion

Q194. A patient collapses during exercise and is found to have hypertrophic cardiomyopathy. What is the most common cause of sudden death in this condition?
(A) Stroke
(B) Valve stenosis
(C) Ventricular arrhythmia
(D) Myocardial rupture

Q195. A patient with chronic renal failure develops elevated potassium and peaked T waves. What is the first medication given to stabilize cardiac membranes?
(A) Calcium gluconate
(B) Furosemide
(C) Insulin
(D) Sodium bicarbonate

Q196. A patient with right-sided heart failure reports abdominal swelling and discomfort. What explains this symptom?
(A) Hepatic congestion from venous backup
(B) Decreased systemic pressure
(C) Reduced renal blood flow only
(D) Increased pulmonary pressure

Q197. A patient with unstable angina shows no improvement despite medication. What is the rationale for early invasive strategy?
(A) Reduce hemoglobin
(B) Identify and treat critical coronary stenosis
(C) Enhance diuresis
(D) Increase heart rate

Q198. A patient with advanced heart failure presents with cold clammy skin and elevated lactate levels. What does elevated lactate signify?
(A) Hyperventilation
(B) Decreased glucose levels
(C) Anaerobic metabolism from hypoperfusion
(D) Improved oxygen delivery

Q199. A patient with atrial flutter has ventricular rate of 150 bpm with 2:1 conduction. What is the typical atrial rate?
(A) 100 bpm
(B) 300 bpm
(C) 75 bpm
(D) 60 bpm

Q200. A patient with massive pulmonary embolism develops hypotension and syncope. What is the immediate life-threatening mechanism?
(A) Left ventricular hypertrophy

(B) Acute right ventricular failure reducing cardiac output
(C) Hypervolemia
(D) Mitral valve prolapse

Answer Key and Explanation (101-200)

Q101. Answer: A

Explanation: Afterload represents the resistance the ventricle must overcome to eject blood. When systemic vascular resistance increases, the heart must generate greater pressure to open the aortic valve. In systolic dysfunction, the weakened myocardium cannot overcome this resistance effectively. As a result, stroke volume decreases and cardiac output falls. Reducing afterload improves forward flow and overall hemodynamics.

Q102. Answer: D

Explanation: Mitral stenosis obstructs blood flow from the left atrium to the left ventricle. This causes persistent elevation of left atrial pressure. Over time, the atrium dilates due to volume and pressure overload. Structural remodeling disrupts normal electrical conduction pathways. These changes predispose the patient to atrial fibrillation.

Q103. Answer: A

Explanation: Beta-blockers reduce sympathetic stimulation of the heart. This lowers heart rate and myocardial contractility. Reduced oxygen demand limits ischemic injury to surrounding myocardium. They also decrease risk of malignant arrhythmias. Long-term therapy improves survival and reduces reinfarction risk.

Q104. Answer: C

Explanation: Right-sided heart failure impairs forward flow into pulmonary circulation. Blood backs up into systemic venous circulation. Elevated venous pressure forces fluid into interstitial tissues. This leads to dependent edema, hepatomegaly, and jugular venous distension. The mechanism is primarily systemic congestion.

Q105. Answer: C

Explanation: Pulmonary edema results from elevated left-sided filling pressures. Diuretics remove excess fluid from circulation. Reduced volume lowers venous return to the heart. This decreases pulmonary capillary pressure. Improved fluid balance enhances gas exchange and symptom relief.

Q106. Answer: D

Explanation: Troponin is a regulatory protein found primarily in cardiac muscle. Its release into circulation indicates myocardial cell damage. Skeletal muscle injury does not significantly elevate cardiac-specific troponin. This specificity reduces false-positive results. Therefore, it is preferred for diagnosing myocardial infarction.

Q107. Answer: A

Explanation: When lying flat, venous return from lower extremities increases. In heart failure, the left ventricle cannot handle the extra volume. Fluid shifts into pulmonary circulation. This worsens congestion and dyspnea. Sitting upright reduces venous return and relieves symptoms.

Q108. Answer: C

Explanation: Potassium plays a key role in maintaining resting membrane potential. Elevated serum potassium decreases the difference between resting and threshold potentials. This disrupts normal depolarization and repolarization cycles. Electrical instability increases arrhythmia risk. Severe elevations may lead to cardiac arrest.

Q109. Answer: D

Explanation: Atrial fibrillation eliminates coordinated atrial contraction. Blood pools within the atrial chambers, especially the left atrial appendage. Stasis promotes thrombus formation. Anticoagulation reduces risk of clot development. This significantly lowers incidence of embolic stroke.

Q110. Answer: C

Explanation: Aortic stenosis narrows the outflow tract from the left ventricle. The heart must generate higher pressure to eject blood. Chronic pressure overload stimulates myocardial fiber thickening. This results in concentric hypertrophy. Initially compensatory, it eventually impairs diastolic filling.

Q111. Answer: C

Explanation: An S3 sound occurs during early diastole. In systolic heart failure, the ventricle is dilated and volume overloaded. Rapid inflow of blood creates vibrations in ventricular walls. This produces the characteristic sound. It often indicates worsening heart failure in adults.

Q112. Answer: B

Explanation: Angiotensin II promotes vasoconstriction and myocardial remodeling. ACE inhibitors block its formation. This reduces pathological structural changes in the ventricle. Limiting remodeling preserves cardiac function. Long-term therapy improves survival outcomes.

Q113. Answer: A

Explanation: Cardiac tamponade involves fluid accumulation in the pericardial sac. External pressure compresses cardiac chambers. Ventricular filling during diastole is restricted. Reduced preload leads to decreased stroke volume. This results in hypotension and shock if untreated.

Q114. Answer: C

Explanation: Organs adapt to chronically elevated blood pressure. Sudden rapid reduction can impair autoregulation. This may cause ischemia in brain, heart, or kidneys. Controlled reduction prevents hypoperfusion injury. Careful titration ensures safe management.

Q115. Answer: D

Explanation: Venous insufficiency results from incompetent valves. Blood pools in lower extremities. Compression stockings apply external pressure to veins. This enhances venous return toward the heart. Reduced pooling decreases edema and ulcer formation.

Q116. Answer: B

Explanation: Hemoglobin carries oxygen to tissues. Low hemoglobin levels reduce oxygen delivery. The heart compensates by increasing cardiac output. Increased workload may provoke ischemia in susceptible individuals. Correction of anemia decreases cardiac strain.

Q117. Answer: A

Explanation: Nitrates primarily cause venous dilation. Reduced venous return decreases left ventricular filling pressure. Lower preload decreases myocardial oxygen demand. Improved oxygen balance alleviates angina. Coronary dilation may also contribute to symptom relief.

Q118. Answer: B

Explanation: A pulmonary embolus blocks blood flow in pulmonary arteries. Gas exchange becomes impaired due to ventilation-perfusion mismatch. Oxygen levels drop rapidly. The patient experiences sudden shortness of breath. Severe obstruction can lead to hemodynamic instability.

Q119. Answer: D

Explanation: Statins reduce hepatic cholesterol synthesis. Lower LDL levels slow progression of atherosclerosis. They also stabilize existing plaques by reducing inflammation. Stable plaques are less likely to rupture. This decreases risk of myocardial infarction and stroke.

Q120. Answer: A

Explanation: Left ventricular failure increases left atrial pressure. Elevated pressure is transmitted backward into pulmonary veins. Persistent elevation raises pulmonary arterial pressures. Over time, pulmonary hypertension develops. This may eventually strain the right ventricle.

Q121. Answer: B

Explanation: ST elevation in anterior leads indicates anterior wall myocardial infarction. The anterior wall involves the left ventricle, which is responsible for systemic circulation. Crackles suggest pulmonary congestion from impaired left ventricular function. Hypotension reflects reduced cardiac output. Acute left ventricular failure is a common and serious complication in this setting.

Q122. Answer: A

Explanation: Atrial fibrillation causes ineffective atrial contraction leading to blood stasis. Clot formation can occur in the atria. Discontinuation of anticoagulation increases embolic risk. An embolus traveling to cerebral circulation can cause sudden neurological deficits. This represents an ischemic stroke due to systemic embolization.

Q123. Answer: A

Explanation: A pulsatile mass at an arterial access site suggests pseudoaneurysm formation. This occurs when blood leaks from the artery but is contained by surrounding tissue. It maintains communication with the arterial lumen. Swelling and localized pain are common findings. Prompt ultrasound evaluation is required.

Q124. Answer: C

Explanation: The presentation strongly suggests acute aortic dissection. Unequal blood pressures and tearing pain are classic findings. Rapid blood pressure control reduces shear stress on the aortic wall. Beta-blockers decrease heart rate and contractility, lowering force on the vessel. Immediate stabilization is essential before surgical evaluation.

Q125. Answer: A

Explanation: When supine, venous return increases from the lower extremities. In heart failure, the left ventricle cannot accommodate the additional volume. Fluid accumulates in pulmonary vasculature. This worsens dyspnea and produces orthopnea. Elevating the head reduces venous return and improves symptoms.

Q126. Answer: B

Explanation: Vegetations on infected valves can break off and travel through systemic circulation. Emboli may lodge in renal arteries. This leads to infarction, flank pain, and hematuria. It is a known complication of infective endocarditis. Rapid diagnosis prevents further organ damage.

Q127. Answer: C

Explanation: Aortic stenosis limits blood ejection from the left ventricle. During exertion, cardiac output cannot increase adequately. Cerebral blood flow decreases transiently. This results in syncope. It is a classic symptom of severe aortic stenosis.

Q128. Answer: C

Explanation: A large pulmonary embolus blocks blood flow in pulmonary arteries. Right ventricular strain increases while left ventricular filling decreases. Reduced cardiac output leads to hypotension. Confusion results from decreased cerebral perfusion. This represents massive pulmonary embolism with hemodynamic instability.

Q129. Answer: C

Explanation: Hypokalemia enhances digoxin binding to myocardial receptors. This increases risk of toxicity. Symptoms include gastrointestinal distress and visual disturbances. Cardiac arrhythmias are common. Monitoring potassium levels reduces risk.

Q130. Answer: C

Explanation: Diminished pulses indicate compromised arterial flow. In diabetes, atherosclerosis commonly affects peripheral arteries. Reduced oxygen delivery delays wound healing. Ischemic ulcers typically occur on toes or pressure points. Vascular assessment is essential.

Q131. Answer: A

Explanation: Papillary muscles support mitral valve function. Infarction may cause rupture leading to acute mitral regurgitation. Blood flows backward into the left atrium during systole. This causes pulmonary edema and dyspnea. It is a life-threatening emergency requiring urgent intervention.

Q132. Answer: A

Explanation: Cardiogenic shock results from pump failure. Increasing myocardial contractility improves cardiac output. Inotropic agents enhance stroke volume. Improved perfusion restores organ function. Close monitoring is required due to arrhythmia risk.

Q133. Answer: B

Explanation: Inferior infarctions may involve the vagus nerve. Enhanced parasympathetic activity slows heart rate. Reduced heart rate lowers cardiac output. Hypotension may result. Atropine can counteract excessive vagal stimulation.

Q134. Answer: D

Explanation: Chronic hypertension increases afterload. The left ventricle adapts by thickening its muscle fibers. This compensatory hypertrophy maintains cardiac output initially. Over time, stiffness impairs filling. Persistent pressure overload leads to heart failure.

Q135. Answer: A

Explanation: Rapid weight gain indicates fluid retention. Adjusting diuretic therapy can prevent worsening congestion. Early intervention reduces hospitalizations. Monitoring daily weight is essential in heart failure management. Prompt action prevents decompensation.

Q136. Answer: B

Explanation: Chaotic irregular waveform without organized complexes indicates ventricular fibrillation. The ventricles quiver ineffectively. Cardiac output ceases immediately. Immediate defibrillation is required. Delay results in death.

Q137. Answer: A

Explanation: Anemia decreases hemoglobin concentration. Oxygen delivery to tissues is reduced. The myocardium becomes ischemic under stress. Coronary disease further limits supply. Correction of anemia alleviates symptoms.

Q138. Answer: A

Explanation: Pulmonary hypertension increases pressure in pulmonary arteries. The right ventricle must pump against higher resistance. Chronic strain leads to right-sided heart failure. Systemic congestion results in edema and liver enlargement. Early management reduces progression.

Q139. Answer: B

Explanation: Persistent chest pain at rest indicates high-risk unstable angina. Medical therapy may not be sufficient. Coronary angiography identifies obstructive lesions. Revascularization may be required. Early invasive strategy improves outcomes.

Q140. Answer: C

Explanation: Large myocardial infarction can severely impair contractility. Reduced cardiac output leads to systemic hypoperfusion. Cool clammy skin reflects vasoconstriction. Hypotension and confusion indicate poor cerebral blood flow. Immediate hemodynamic support is necessary.

Q141. Answer: B

Explanation: Chronic left ventricular dysfunction increases pulmonary pressures over time. Elevated pulmonary resistance places strain on the right ventricle. Eventually, right ventricular failure develops, leading to systemic venous congestion. Jugular venous distension and hepatomegaly reflect backward pressure in systemic circulation. This progression is common in advanced heart failure.

Q142. Answer: D

Explanation: Patients with renal failure are prone to potassium imbalance. Elevated potassium levels alter cardiac conduction. Peaked T waves are characteristic ECG findings. Severe hyperkalemia may lead to arrhythmias and hypotension. Prompt correction is essential to prevent cardiac arrest.

Q143. Answer: D

Explanation: Atrial fibrillation predisposes to thrombus formation. Embolization can occur to mesenteric arteries. Sudden severe abdominal pain with minimal findings suggests ischemia. Bowel sounds may be reduced due to infarction. Immediate intervention is required to prevent bowel necrosis.

Q144. Answer: B

Explanation: Post-infarction pericarditis can occur days after myocardial injury. Inflammation of the pericardium causes pleuritic chest pain. Positional relief when leaning forward is characteristic. It differs from ischemic pain in quality and timing. Anti-inflammatory treatment is usually effective.

Q145. Answer: B

Explanation: Chronic hypertension weakens small cerebral vessels. Persistent high pressure leads to microaneurysm formation. Vessel rupture results in intracerebral hemorrhage. Sudden neurological deficits are typical. Blood pressure control is critical for prevention.

Q146. Answer: D

Explanation: Stable angina results from fixed atherosclerotic narrowing. At rest, coronary perfusion meets myocardial demand. During exertion, oxygen demand exceeds supply. This imbalance produces chest pain. Rest reduces workload and restores balance.

Q147. Answer: D

Explanation: Excessive fluid administration may overwhelm cardiac function. Increased hydrostatic pressure in pulmonary capillaries causes fluid leakage. Crackles and hypoxia suggest pulmonary edema. Patients with limited cardiac reserve are especially vulnerable. Fluid management must be carefully balanced.

Q148. Answer: B

Explanation: Mitral regurgitation increases blood volume returning to the left atrium. Chronic overload leads to atrial enlargement. Structural remodeling disrupts electrical conduction pathways. This predisposes to atrial fibrillation. Early valve repair may reduce long-term complications.

Q149. Answer: D

Explanation: Pulseless ventricular tachycardia is treated like ventricular fibrillation. Immediate unsynchronized defibrillation is required. Delayed treatment reduces survival. High-quality CPR should accompany resuscitation efforts. Early shock delivery is critical.

Q150. Answer: C

Explanation: Severe hypotension with signs of end-organ hypoperfusion indicates shock. Reduced cardiac output leads to decreased renal perfusion. Confusion reflects cerebral hypoxia. This represents decompensated cardiogenic shock. Immediate circulatory support is required.

Q151. Answer: A

Explanation: Painless lesions on palms and soles suggest embolic phenomena. Fragments from infected valve vegetations can travel through circulation. These cause small vascular occlusions. They are characteristic of systemic embolization. Prompt antibiotic therapy is essential.

Q152. Answer: D

Explanation: Peripheral arterial disease limits blood flow to muscles. During walking, oxygen demand increases. Narrowed arteries cannot meet demand. Temporary ischemia causes cramping pain. Rest restores oxygen balance and relieves symptoms.

Q153. Answer: D

Explanation: Advanced renal failure leads to accumulation of uremic toxins. These irritate the pericardial lining. Inflammation causes friction rub and chest discomfort. This condition is common in untreated uremia. Dialysis often improves symptoms.

Q154. Answer: D

Explanation: Prosthetic valves increase risk of infection. Bacteremia can seed artificial surfaces. Fever and positive cultures suggest infective endocarditis. Early diagnosis is critical due to high mortality. Aggressive antibiotic therapy is required.

Q155. Answer: A

Explanation: Obstruction of pulmonary artery branches reduces blood supply to lung tissue. Prolonged obstruction may cause infarction. Tissue necrosis can lead to hemoptysis. Pleuritic pain occurs from inflammation of pleural surfaces. Rapid anticoagulation limits progression.

Q156. Answer: C

Explanation: Diabetes can damage autonomic nerves. Impaired nerve function reduces perception of ischemic pain. Myocardial infarction may occur without classic symptoms. This increases risk of delayed treatment. High suspicion is needed in diabetic patients.

Q157. Answer: A

Explanation: Severe heart failure reduces cardiac output. Circulatory delay affects carbon dioxide sensing in brainstem. This leads to cyclical breathing patterns. Periods of apnea alternate with hyperventilation. It reflects advanced cardiac dysfunction.

Q158. Answer: B

Explanation: A thrombus in deep veins can dislodge. Embolization to pulmonary arteries impairs circulation. Sudden hypotension and tachycardia indicate hemodynamic compromise. This is a medical emergency. Rapid treatment improves survival.

Q159. Answer: C

Explanation: Cardiomyopathy often leads to myocardial fibrosis. Scar tissue disrupts normal conduction pathways. Abnormal circuits predispose to reentrant arrhythmias. Sustained ventricular tachycardia may occur. Implantable defibrillator therapy may be indicated.

Q160. Answer: D

Explanation: Chest trauma may cause bleeding into pericardial sac. Fluid accumulation compresses the heart. Impaired filling reduces cardiac output. Distended neck veins reflect elevated venous pressure. Clear lungs help differentiate from pulmonary edema. Immediate pericardiocentesis is required.

Q161. Answer: A

Explanation: Chest pain at rest with ST depression suggests acute coronary syndrome. Elevated troponin confirms myocardial injury without ST elevation. This pattern is consistent with non-ST elevation myocardial infarction. It indicates partial coronary artery occlusion. Early antiplatelet and anticoagulant therapy are essential to limit further damage.

Q162. Answer: C

Explanation: Diuretics remove sodium and water from circulation. Excessive dosing may lead to hypovolemia. Reduced circulating volume lowers blood pressure. Decreased preload may also reduce cardiac output. Careful titration is required to avoid symptomatic hypotension.

Q163. Answer: A

Explanation: Ascending aortic dissection is a surgical emergency. The tear in the aorta can rapidly lead to rupture or organ ischemia. Medical therapy may stabilize blood pressure temporarily. Definitive management requires surgical repair. Early intervention significantly improves survival.

Q164. Answer: C

Explanation: Persistent rapid ventricular rates reduce diastolic filling time. Chronic tachycardia strains the myocardium. Over time, ventricular function declines. This condition is known as tachycardia-induced cardiomyopathy. Rate control is essential to reverse dysfunction.

Q165. Answer: B

Explanation: Ventricular septal rupture is a mechanical complication of myocardial infarction. It creates abnormal blood flow between ventricles. The resulting murmur is typically harsh and holosystolic. Hypotension occurs due to reduced effective cardiac output. Immediate surgical consultation is required.

Q166. Answer: B

Explanation: A portion of the thrombus may have embolized before full anticoagulation effect. Pulmonary embolism presents with acute chest pain and dyspnea. Rapid evaluation is required. Imaging confirms diagnosis. Prompt management reduces mortality.

Q167. Answer: C

Explanation: Hypertrophic cardiomyopathy involves dynamic outflow obstruction. Reduced preload decreases ventricular chamber size. This worsens obstruction of blood flow. Vasodilators lower preload and may intensify symptoms. Careful medication selection is necessary.

Q168. Answer: D

Explanation: The findings represent cardiac tamponade. Accumulated fluid compresses the heart. Ventricular filling is severely restricted. Immediate drainage of pericardial fluid restores cardiac output. Delayed treatment may be fatal.

Q169. Answer: D

Explanation: Anemia reduces oxygen-carrying capacity. The heart compensates by increasing cardiac output. Persistent overwork strains myocardial function. Over time, heart failure symptoms may develop. Correction of anemia improves cardiac workload.

Q170. Answer: D

Explanation: Uremic toxins accumulate in advanced kidney disease. These toxins irritate the pericardium. Inflammation may lead to fluid accumulation. Pericardial effusion can impair cardiac function. Dialysis often alleviates symptoms.

Q171. Answer: A

Explanation: Pulmonary embolism increases pulmonary vascular resistance. The right ventricle struggles against this sudden pressure load. Right-sided pressures rise. This leads to jugular venous distension. Clear lungs help distinguish from left-sided failure.

Q172. Answer: B

Explanation: Concentric hypertrophy thickens ventricular walls. This reduces compliance. Impaired relaxation limits diastolic filling. Diastolic dysfunction may lead to heart failure with preserved ejection fraction. Long-term blood pressure control is essential.

Q173. Answer: B

Explanation: Central venous catheter use can cause lung puncture. Air enters pleural space. Collapsed lung reduces oxygenation. Hypotension may occur with tension physiology. Immediate decompression is required.

Q174. Answer: B

Explanation: During sleep, fluid from peripheral tissues returns to circulation. Increased preload overwhelms failing ventricle. Pulmonary congestion worsens at night. Sudden awakening with dyspnea occurs. Sitting upright relieves symptoms.

Q175. Answer: B

Explanation: Vegetations contain bacteria and fibrin. Small fragments may embolize to peripheral vessels. Capillary damage causes linear hemorrhages under nails. These findings support systemic embolization. Early antibiotic therapy is critical.

Q176. Answer: B

Explanation: Asystole is a non-shockable rhythm. Defibrillation is not effective. Immediate CPR maintains circulation. Epinephrine supports perfusion pressure. Rapid intervention is vital for survival.

Q177. Answer: D

Explanation: Mitral stenosis elevates left atrial pressure. This pressure transmits backward to pulmonary veins. Increased capillary pressure may cause rupture of small vessels. Hemoptysis can result. It reflects advanced pulmonary congestion.

Q178. Answer: D

Explanation: Severely reduced ejection fraction increases arrhythmia risk. Implantable defibrillators detect and treat life-threatening rhythms. They reduce sudden cardiac death. Device therapy is recommended in selected patients. Survival improves with appropriate selection.

Q179. Answer: D

Explanation: Inferior wall infarctions may stimulate the vagus nerve. Increased parasympathetic activity causes bradycardia and nausea. Hypotension may result from decreased heart rate. These features are characteristic of inferior infarcts. Recognition guides management.

Q180. Answer: A

Explanation: Poor cardiac output reduces tissue oxygenation. Cells switch to anaerobic metabolism. Lactate accumulates as a byproduct. Elevated lactate indicates inadequate perfusion. Improving circulation corrects metabolic acidosis.

Q181. Answer: C

Explanation: Pink frothy sputum indicates acute pulmonary edema. Elevated blood pressure increases hydrostatic pressure in pulmonary capillaries. Oxygen improves gas exchange while diuretics reduce intravascular volume. Rapid preload reduction decreases pulmonary congestion. Early treatment prevents respiratory failure.

Q182. Answer: A

Explanation: Atrial fibrillation predisposes to clot formation in the atria. Interrupting anticoagulation increases embolic risk. Surgery requires balancing bleeding and clotting risks. Bridging strategies may be used in high-risk individuals. Careful planning minimizes complications.

Q183. Answer: B

Explanation: Aortic regurgitation causes blood to flow back into the left ventricle during diastole. This increases stroke volume and systolic pressure. Diastolic pressure falls due to regurgitation. The result is widened pulse pressure. Peripheral signs reflect this hemodynamic pattern.

Q184. Answer: D

Explanation: Large myocardial infarction can severely impair contractility. Reduced cardiac output leads to systemic hypoperfusion. Confusion and low urine output reflect end-organ dysfunction. Hypotension indicates failure of compensatory mechanisms. Immediate circulatory support is required.

Q185. Answer: B

Explanation: Diffuse ST elevation with PR depression is characteristic of pericarditis. Unlike STEMI, changes are not localized to a coronary territory. Normal troponin suggests absence of significant myocardial necrosis. Inflammation of the pericardium causes these ECG findings. Anti-inflammatory therapy is commonly used.

Q186. Answer: A

Explanation: Dilated cardiomyopathy impairs forward cardiac output. Blood backs up into systemic circulation. Elevated venous pressure pushes fluid into interstitial spaces. This results in edema and ascites. Management focuses on improving cardiac function and reducing volume overload.

Q187. Answer: C

Explanation: Anticoagulants prevent extension of existing thrombus. They reduce risk of additional embolic events. Clot dissolution occurs gradually through natural fibrinolysis. Preventing propagation decreases mortality risk. Early initiation is critical.

Q188. Answer: A

Explanation: Thickened ventricular walls reduce compliance. Impaired relaxation limits diastolic filling. Ejection fraction remains preserved. This pattern is consistent with heart failure with preserved ejection fraction. Hypertension is a common underlying cause.

Q189. Answer: C

Explanation: Thrombolytics increase bleeding risk. Sudden neurological symptoms suggest intracranial bleeding. This is a life-threatening complication. Immediate discontinuation and evaluation are required. Early detection improves survival.

Q190. Answer: A

Explanation: Pale, cool extremities with delayed capillary refill indicate severe arterial insufficiency. Reduced blood flow compromises tissue viability. Numbness suggests nerve ischemia. Without intervention, tissue necrosis may occur. Urgent vascular assessment is necessary.

Q191. Answer: A

Explanation: Severe valve destruction impairs normal blood flow. Regurgitation or obstruction increases cardiac workload. Rapid decompensation can occur. Acute heart failure develops if structural damage persists. Surgical intervention may be required.

Q192. Answer: C

Explanation: Wide complex tachycardia often indicates ventricular origin. In heart failure, myocardial scarring predisposes to ventricular arrhythmias. Sustained ventricular tachycardia can compromise perfusion. Immediate assessment and treatment are necessary. Risk of progression to cardiac arrest exists.

Q193. Answer: D

Explanation: Mitral stenosis elevates left atrial pressure. Backward transmission increases pulmonary venous pressure. Capillary rupture may cause hemoptysis. Pulmonary congestion leads to dyspnea. Chronic elevation can cause pulmonary hypertension.

Q194. Answer: C

Explanation: Hypertrophic cardiomyopathy disrupts normal myocardial structure. Electrical instability predisposes to lethal arrhythmias. Sudden cardiac death often occurs during exertion. Implantable defibrillators reduce risk in high-risk patients. Early detection is vital.

Q195. Answer: A

Explanation: Hyperkalemia affects cardiac conduction. Calcium gluconate stabilizes myocardial cell membranes. It reduces risk of arrhythmias rapidly. It does not lower potassium levels but buys time for definitive treatment. Continuous ECG monitoring is necessary.

Q196. Answer: A

Explanation: Right-sided heart failure causes systemic venous congestion. Elevated pressure affects abdominal organs. Liver enlargement and ascites may develop. Fluid accumulation produces abdominal discomfort. Managing venous congestion improves symptoms.

Q197. Answer: B

Explanation: Persistent symptoms indicate ongoing ischemia. Coronary angiography identifies obstructive lesions. Revascularization restores blood flow. Early intervention reduces risk of infarction. Timely management improves prognosis.

Q198. Answer: C

Explanation: Poor perfusion limits oxygen supply to tissues. Cells switch to anaerobic metabolism. Lactate accumulates as a byproduct. Elevated levels indicate severe hypoperfusion. Monitoring trends helps assess response to therapy.

Q199. Answer: B

Explanation: Atrial flutter typically generates atrial rates around 300 beats per minute. With 2:1 conduction, every second impulse reaches the ventricles. This produces a ventricular rate of 150 bpm. The atrial activity appears as sawtooth waves on ECG. Rate control is often necessary.

Q200. Answer: B

Explanation: Massive pulmonary embolism suddenly increases pulmonary vascular resistance. The right ventricle cannot overcome the obstruction. Cardiac output drops dramatically. Hypotension and syncope occur due to reduced cerebral perfusion. Immediate aggressive management is critical to survival.

Question (201-300)

Q201. A 58-year-old male with a history of hypertension presents with sudden onset tearing chest pain radiating to the back and unequal blood pressures in both arms. Which is the most likely diagnosis?

(A) Acute pericarditis
(B) Pulmonary embolism
(C) Aortic dissection
(D) Unstable angina

Q202. Which electrolyte abnormality is most likely to precipitate ventricular tachycardia in a patient on digoxin therapy?

(A) Hypokalemia
(B) Hyponatremia
(C) Hypercalcemia
(D) Hyperkalemia

Q203. A patient with heart failure reports waking at night short of breath and needing to sit upright to breathe comfortably. This symptom is known as:

(A) Orthopnea
(B) Exertional dyspnea
(C) Cheyne-Stokes respiration
(D) Paroxysmal nocturnal dyspnea

Q204. Which medication class has been shown to reduce mortality in patients with systolic heart failure?

(A) Calcium channel blockers
(B) ACE inhibitors
(C) Loop diuretics
(D) Nitrates alone

Q205. A patient presents with crushing substernal chest pain lasting 30 minutes and ST elevation in leads II, III, and aVF. Which coronary artery is most likely involved?

(A) Right coronary artery
(B) Left circumflex artery
(C) Left anterior descending artery
(D) Diagonal branch

Q206. Which finding is most characteristic of cardiac tamponade?

(A) Beck's triad
(B) Bounding pulses
(C) Widened pulse pressure
(D) Loud S1

Q207. A patient with atrial fibrillation is at greatest risk for which complication?

(A) Stroke
(B) Ventricular septal defect
(C) Endocarditis
(D) Pulmonary hypertension

Q208. Which heart sound is associated with rapid ventricular filling and is commonly heard in heart failure?

(A) S2
(B) S3
(C) S1
(D) S4

Q209. A patient taking warfarin has an INR of 6.5 without bleeding. The most appropriate intervention is:

(A) Administer thrombolytics
(B) Increase warfarin dose
(C) Hold warfarin and monitor
(D) Start heparin

Q210. Which condition is most strongly associated with a harsh systolic murmur radiating to the carotids?

(A) Tricuspid regurgitation
(B) Aortic stenosis
(C) Mitral regurgitation
(D) Pulmonary stenosis

Q211. The primary mechanism of action of beta-blockers in ischemic heart disease is:

(A) Enhancing platelet aggregation
(B) Decreasing myocardial oxygen demand
(C) Increasing preload
(D) Increasing coronary vasodilation

Q212. A patient develops sudden dyspnea and pleuritic chest pain after prolonged immobilization. Which diagnostic test is most appropriate initially?

(A) CT pulmonary angiography
(B) Echocardiogram
(C) Cardiac catheterization
(D) Exercise stress test

Q213. Which medication is first-line for rate control in stable atrial fibrillation?

(A) Adenosine
(B) Epinephrine
(C) Atropine
(D) Metoprolol

Q214. A widened pulse pressure is most commonly seen in:
(A) Pulmonary embolism
(B) Aortic regurgitation
(C) Cardiac tamponade
(D) Mitral stenosis
Q215. Which lab marker rises earliest after myocardial infarction?
(A) Troponin
(B) CK-MB
(C) Myoglobin
(D) BNP
Q216. Which intervention is most appropriate for symptomatic bradycardia with hypotension?
(A) Amiodarone
(B) Atropine
(C) Magnesium sulfate
(D) Lidocaine
Q217. Which lifestyle modification most effectively reduces cardiovascular risk in smokers?
(A) Daily vitamin supplementation
(B) Reducing caffeine intake
(C) Smoking cessation
(D) Increased protein intake
Q218. Which condition is characterized by electrical activity without a palpable pulse?
(A) Asystole
(B) Atrial flutter
(C) Pulseless electrical activity
(D) Ventricular fibrillation
Q219. Which diagnostic finding confirms infective endocarditis?
(A) Elevated ESR
(B) Positive blood cultures
(C) Chest pain
(D) Tachycardia
Q220. Which medication is indicated to reduce preload in acute pulmonary edema?
(A) Warfarin
(B) Digoxin
(C) Furosemide
(D) Dopamine
Q221. A 65-year-old woman presents with progressive exertional dyspnea and a mid-diastolic murmur best heard at the apex with the patient in the left lateral position. What is the most likely diagnosis?
(A) Tricuspid stenosis
(B) Mitral stenosis
(C) Mitral regurgitation
(D) Aortic stenosis
Q222. A patient with left-sided heart failure most commonly develops which complication?
(A) Hepatomegaly
(B) Pulmonary congestion
(C) Ascites
(D) Peripheral edema
Q223. Which antiarrhythmic medication is most appropriate for treating stable ventricular tachycardia?
(A) Verapamil
(B) Atropine
(C) Amiodarone
(D) Adenosine
Q224. Which condition is characterized by chest pain that improves when leaning forward?
(A) Myocardial infarction
(B) Stable angina
(C) Acute pericarditis
(D) Pulmonary embolism
Q225. Which laboratory value is most useful in diagnosing heart failure exacerbation?
(A) Creatinine
(B) Hemoglobin
(C) Troponin
(D) BNP
Q226. A patient with hypertrophic cardiomyopathy is at increased risk for:
(A) Sudden cardiac death
(B) Infective endocarditis only
(C) Pulmonary fibrosis
(D) Aortic dissection
Q227. Which intervention is most appropriate in pulseless ventricular fibrillation?
(A) Adenosine injection
(B) Immediate defibrillation
(C) Atropine administration
(D) Synchronized cardioversion
Q228. A patient presents with unilateral leg swelling and pain. Which condition should be suspected to prevent pulmonary embolism?
(A) Deep vein thrombosis

(B) Cellulitis
(C) Peripheral artery disease
(D) Lymphedema

Q229. Which finding is most consistent with right-sided heart failure?
(A) Jugular venous distension
(B) S3 at apex
(C) Orthopnea
(D) Crackles in lungs

Q230. Which drug reduces platelet aggregation by inhibiting the P2Y12 receptor?
(A) Warfarin
(B) Aspirin
(C) Clopidogrel
(D) Heparin

Q231. A patient with severe aortic stenosis most likely experiences which symptom?
(A) Cyanosis at birth
(B) Hemoptysis
(C) Polyuria
(D) Syncope during exertion

Q232. Which ECG change is most specific for acute myocardial infarction?
(A) Premature atrial contractions
(B) Sinus tachycardia
(C) First-degree AV block
(D) ST elevation in contiguous leads

Q233. Which medication is contraindicated in patients taking nitrates for angina?
(A) Sildenafil
(B) Statins
(C) Beta-blockers
(D) ACE inhibitors

Q234. Which parameter is most useful in assessing anticoagulation with heparin?
(A) INR
(B) aPTT
(C) Platelet count
(D) D-dimer

Q235. A patient presents with chest pain and diffuse ST elevation with PR depression on ECG. What is the most likely diagnosis?
(A) Acute pericarditis
(B) STEMI
(C) Aortic aneurysm
(D) Unstable angina

Q236. Which condition is associated with a loud S4 heart sound?
(A) Dilated cardiomyopathy
(B) Ventricular hypertrophy
(C) Atrial septal defect
(D) Acute mitral regurgitation

Q237. Which lipid abnormality is most strongly linked to atherosclerosis?
(A) Elevated LDL
(B) Low triglycerides
(C) Elevated HDL
(D) Low total cholesterol

Q238. Which is the first-line therapy for anaphylaxis with cardiovascular collapse?
(A) Epinephrine
(B) Diphenhydramine
(C) Hydrocortisone
(D) Albuterol

Q239. A patient with chronic hypertension is at risk for which structural cardiac change?
(A) Left ventricular hypertrophy
(B) Patent ductus arteriosus
(C) Ventricular septal defect
(D) Right atrial enlargement

Q240. Which intervention improves survival in patients after myocardial infarction?
(A) Routine antiarrhythmic prophylaxis
(B) Long-term oxygen therapy
(C) Bed rest for 6 weeks
(D) Early beta-blocker therapy

Q241. A patient with acute anterior myocardial infarction develops hypotension, clear lung fields, and elevated jugular venous pressure. Which complication is most likely?
(A) Papillary muscle rupture
(B) Ventricular septal rupture
(C) Right ventricular infarction
(D) Left ventricular failure

Q242. Which medication is most appropriate to relieve acute angina pain?
(A) Sublingual nitroglycerin
(B) Atorvastatin
(C) Digoxin
(D) Furosemide

Q243. A patient with infective endocarditis is at highest risk for which systemic complication?
(A) Chronic bronchitis
(B) Peptic ulcer disease
(C) Pulmonary fibrosis

(D) Embolic stroke

Q244. Which finding indicates worsening left ventricular systolic dysfunction?

(A) Reduced cardiac output
(B) Narrow pulse pressure
(C) Decreased BNP
(D) Increased ejection fraction

Q245. A continuous "machinery-like" murmur is characteristic of which condition?

(A) Atrial septal defect
(B) Mitral valve prolapse
(C) Ventricular septal defect
(D) Patent ductus arteriosus

Q246. Which medication is most associated with development of a persistent dry cough?

(A) Lisinopril
(B) Metoprolol
(C) Losartan
(D) Amlodipine

Q247. A patient with severe mitral regurgitation is most likely to develop which chamber enlargement?

(A) Left atrium
(B) Pulmonary artery
(C) Right ventricle
(D) Right atrium

Q248. Which rhythm is characterized by irregularly irregular R-R intervals without distinct P waves?

(A) Sinus arrhythmia
(B) Atrial flutter
(C) Atrial fibrillation
(D) Ventricular tachycardia

Q249. Which condition is most associated with pulsus paradoxus?

(A) Aortic stenosis
(B) Hyperlipidemia
(C) Hypertension
(D) Cardiac tamponade

Q250. Which drug class decreases mortality in patients with reduced ejection fraction heart failure?

(A) Thiazide diuretics
(B) Beta-blockers
(C) Calcium channel blockers
(D) Nitrates alone

Q251. A patient develops sudden severe chest pain and shortness of breath after central line placement. Which complication is most likely?

(A) Myocardial infarction
(B) Pericarditis
(C) Endocarditis
(D) Pneumothorax

Q252. Which biomarker is most specific for myocardial necrosis?

(A) LDH
(B) Myoglobin
(C) CK-MB
(D) Troponin I

Q253. A patient with uncontrolled hypertension presents with headache, visual changes, and BP 220/120 mmHg. This condition is best described as:

(A) Orthostatic hypotension
(B) Hypertensive urgency
(C) Hypertensive emergency
(D) White coat hypertension

Q254. Which condition most commonly leads to secondary hypertension?

(A) Renal artery stenosis
(B) Sedentary lifestyle
(C) Hyperlipidemia
(D) Essential hypertension

Q255. Which intervention is most important in preventing deep vein thrombosis in hospitalized patients?

(A) Fluid restriction
(B) High-fat diet
(C) Strict bed rest
(D) Early ambulation

Q256. A patient with atrial flutter typically demonstrates which ECG pattern?

(A) Irregular baseline without P waves
(B) Prolonged PR interval
(C) Wide QRS complexes
(D) Sawtooth flutter waves

Q257. Which medication is most appropriate for lowering LDL cholesterol?

(A) Niacin
(B) Digoxin
(C) Statin
(D) Fibrate

Q258. Which symptom is most typical of peripheral arterial disease?

(A) Resting leg swelling
(B) Intermittent claudication
(C) Cyanosis at birth
(D) Productive cough

Q259. Which cardiac enzyme remains elevated the longest after myocardial infarction?
(A) Troponin
(B) Myoglobin
(C) AST
(D) CK-MB

Q260. Which condition is characterized by narrowing of the mitral valve opening leading to obstructed left ventricular filling?
(A) Tricuspid regurgitation
(B) Mitral regurgitation
(C) Aortic regurgitation
(D) Mitral stenosis

Q261. A 72-year-old patient with chronic atrial fibrillation suddenly develops right-sided weakness and slurred speech. What is the most likely underlying cause?
(A) Migraine aura
(B) Intracranial hemorrhage
(C) Embolic ischemic stroke
(D) Hypoglycemia

Q262. A patient with acute decompensated heart failure presents with severe dyspnea, pink frothy sputum, and crackles throughout both lung fields. What is the priority intervention?
(A) Place in supine position
(B) Administer IV fluids rapidly
(C) Administer IV loop diuretic
(D) Encourage oral hydration

Q263. A patient with unstable angina continues to have chest pain despite nitrates. Which medication should be administered next to reduce myocardial oxygen demand?
(A) Epinephrine
(B) Dopamine
(C) Atropine
(D) Beta-blocker

Q264. Following cardiac catheterization via the femoral artery, the patient reports severe back pain and hypotension. What complication should be suspected?
(A) Retroperitoneal hemorrhage
(B) Pulmonary embolism
(C) Pericarditis
(D) Aortic stenosis

Q265. A patient with heart failure has gained 3 pounds in 24 hours and reports increasing shortness of breath. What is the most appropriate nursing action?
(A) Discontinue beta-blocker
(B) Increase sodium intake
(C) Notify provider and adjust diuretics
(D) Reassure and schedule follow-up

Q266. A patient receiving heparin therapy develops a platelet count drop of 50% from baseline. What is the most appropriate action?
(A) Administer aspirin
(B) Increase heparin dose
(C) Continue heparin and monitor
(D) Discontinue heparin immediately

Q267. A patient with inferior myocardial infarction becomes bradycardic and hypotensive. Which medication is most appropriate initially?
(A) Lidocaine
(B) Atropine
(C) Amiodarone
(D) Nitroglycerin

Q268. A patient with mechanical heart valve replacement requires long-term therapy with which medication?
(A) Aspirin only
(B) Warfarin
(C) Clopidogrel only
(D) Digoxin

Q269. A patient presents with tearing chest pain and a widened mediastinum on chest X-ray. What is the next best diagnostic test?
(A) Exercise stress test
(B) Holter monitor
(C) Echocardiogram only
(D) CT angiography

Q270. A patient with chronic stable angina wants to prevent future episodes. Which long-term medication is most appropriate?
(A) Long-acting nitrate
(B) Short-acting nitrate only
(C) Thrombolytic agent
(D) Epinephrine

Q271. A patient develops sudden confusion and hypotension after rapid administration of

antihypertensive medication. What is the likely cause?
(A) Reflex hypertension
(B) Hyperglycemia
(C) Cerebral hypoperfusion
(D) Fluid overload

Q272. A patient with dilated cardiomyopathy presents with worsening fatigue and peripheral edema. Which diagnostic test best evaluates ventricular function?
(A) D-dimer
(B) Chest X-ray
(C) ECG
(D) Echocardiogram

Q273. A patient receiving thrombolytic therapy for STEMI develops sudden severe headache. What is the priority action?
(A) Administer aspirin
(B) Continue infusion
(C) Encourage ambulation
(D) Stop infusion and notify provider

Q274. A patient with peripheral arterial disease reports leg pain at rest that improves when dangling legs over the side of the bed. What does this indicate?
(A) Normal aging
(B) Venous insufficiency
(C) Muscle strain
(D) Advanced arterial disease

Q275. A patient presents with acute chest pain and ST elevation in V1-V4. Which region of the heart is affected?
(A) Anterior wall
(B) Lateral wall
(C) Posterior wall
(D) Inferior wall

Q276. A patient with heart failure is prescribed spironolactone. What electrolyte imbalance should be monitored closely?
(A) Hypercalcemia
(B) Hyponatremia
(C) Hypokalemia
(D) Hyperkalemia

Q277. A patient experiences syncope during exertion and is diagnosed with severe aortic stenosis. What is the definitive treatment?
(A) Beta-blocker alone
(B) Valve replacement
(C) Lifestyle modification
(D) Diuretic therapy only

Q278. A hospitalized patient suddenly develops sharp chest pain and shortness of breath after prolonged bed rest. What is the most likely diagnosis?
(A) Pulmonary embolism
(B) Myocarditis
(C) Stable angina
(D) Pericardial effusion

Q279. A patient with uncontrolled diabetes and hypertension presents with chest discomfort. Which risk factor most significantly increases cardiovascular disease progression?
(A) Occasional caffeine intake
(B) Hyperglycemia
(C) Seasonal allergies
(D) Mild dehydration

Q280. A patient recovering from myocardial infarction asks about cardiac rehabilitation. What is the primary benefit of participation?
(A) Avoidance of follow-up visits
(B) Reduced risk of recurrent events
(C) Immediate cure of coronary disease
(D) Elimination of all medications

Q281. A 68-year-old patient with long-standing hypertension presents with progressive shortness of breath and an S4 heart sound. Echocardiogram shows preserved ejection fraction. What is the most likely diagnosis?
(A) Acute myocarditis
(B) Right ventricular infarction
(C) Systolic heart failure
(D) Diastolic heart failure

Q282. A patient receiving IV amiodarone develops hypotension and bradycardia. What is the priority nursing intervention?
(A) Encourage ambulation
(B) Increase infusion rate
(C) Administer potassium
(D) Stop infusion temporarily

Q283. A patient with chest trauma develops muffled heart sounds, distended neck veins, and hypotension. What is the most likely diagnosis?
(A) Tension pneumothorax
(B) Pulmonary edema
(C) Cardiac tamponade

(D) Myocardial contusion

Q284. A patient with chronic atrial fibrillation is not on anticoagulation and presents with sudden abdominal pain. Which complication should be suspected?

(A) Appendicitis
(B) Mesenteric ischemia
(C) Peptic ulcer
(D) Pancreatitis

Q285. A patient with heart failure is instructed to follow a low-sodium diet. What is the primary reason for this recommendation?

(A) Improve oxygen saturation
(B) Reduce fluid retention
(C) Increase heart rate
(D) Prevent arrhythmias

Q286. A patient with severe peripheral arterial disease has a pale, cool foot with diminished pulses. What is the most urgent concern?

(A) Acute limb ischemia
(B) Venous thrombosis
(C) Cellulitis
(D) Lymphedema

Q287. A patient develops new-onset atrial fibrillation with rapid ventricular response and blood pressure of 80/50 mmHg. What is the most appropriate intervention?

(A) Oral beta-blocker
(B) Observation only
(C) Synchronized cardioversion
(D) Aspirin therapy

Q288. A patient taking statins reports muscle pain and weakness. Which laboratory test should be checked?

(A) D-dimer
(B) Hemoglobin
(C) Creatine kinase
(D) Serum potassium

Q289. A patient presents with chest pain relieved by rest and predictable with exertion. What is the most likely diagnosis?

(A) Myocardial infarction
(B) Unstable angina
(C) Stable angina
(D) Variant angina

Q290. A patient with left ventricular failure develops confusion and decreased urine output. What is the underlying cause?

(A) Decreased cardiac output
(B) Hypervolemia
(C) Increased cerebral perfusion
(D) Pulmonary hypertension

Q291. A patient with suspected deep vein thrombosis has a positive D-dimer. What is the next best diagnostic step?

(A) Perform venous ultrasound
(B) Start thrombolytics immediately
(C) Administer aspirin
(D) Order stress test

Q292. A patient with hypertrophic cardiomyopathy collapses during exercise. What is the most likely mechanism?

(A) Hypoglycemia
(B) Ventricular arrhythmia
(C) Dehydration
(D) Pulmonary embolism

Q293. A patient receiving ACE inhibitor therapy develops facial swelling and difficulty breathing. What is the immediate concern?

(A) Dry cough
(B) Hyperkalemia
(C) Angioedema
(D) Hyponatremia

Q294. A patient with chronic venous insufficiency presents with brownish skin discoloration around the ankles. What is the cause?

(A) Acute thrombosis
(B) Cyanosis
(C) Arterial blockage
(D) Hemosiderin deposition

Q295. A patient with acute myocardial infarction develops a new loud holosystolic murmur and pulmonary edema. What complication is suspected?

(A) Pericarditis
(B) Aortic dissection
(C) Ventricular septal rupture
(D) Stable angina

Q296. A patient on long-term warfarin therapy presents with INR of 9 and minor bleeding. What is the most appropriate management?

(A) Administer vitamin K
(B) Discontinue all therapy permanently
(C) Increase warfarin dose
(D) Start heparin

Q297. A patient with severe heart failure is prescribed an implantable cardioverter-defibrillator. What is its primary purpose?
(A) Improve ejection fraction
(B) Eliminate need for medications
(C) Reduce blood pressure
(D) Prevent sudden cardiac death

Q298. A patient presents with fever, new heart murmur, and positive blood cultures. Which diagnostic study best confirms valvular involvement?
(A) Lipid profile
(B) Echocardiography
(C) Chest X-ray
(D) ECG

Q299. A patient with long-standing diabetes complains of numbness in feet and diminished pulses. What complication is most likely?
(A) Diabetic neuropathy with peripheral arterial disease
(B) Acute myocarditis
(C) Pericardial effusion
(D) Atrial septal defect

Q300. A patient recovering from cardiac surgery develops sudden shortness of breath and decreased oxygen saturation. What is the priority assessment?
(A) Measure height and weight
(B) Assess bowel sounds
(C) Check surgical dressing
(D) Auscultate lung sounds

Answer Key and Explanation (201-300)

Q201. Answer: C

Explanation: Sudden tearing chest pain radiating to the back with unequal arm blood pressures strongly suggests acute aortic dissection. The unequal pressures occur due to involvement of major arterial branches from the aorta. This condition is life-threatening and requires immediate imaging and blood pressure control. Pericarditis pain is typically positional and pleuritic. Pulmonary embolism presents more commonly with dyspnea and hypoxia, while unstable angina causes pressure-like chest discomfort without radiation to the back in a tearing pattern.

Q202. Answer: A

Explanation: Hypokalemia increases myocardial sensitivity to digoxin and predisposes patients to ventricular arrhythmias. Low potassium enhances digoxin binding to sodium-potassium ATPase, increasing toxicity risk. Ventricular tachycardia is a known complication in this setting. Hyperkalemia is more often associated with conduction blocks. Hypercalcemia may increase contractility but is less directly linked to digoxin-induced ventricular tachycardia, and hyponatremia does not significantly influence digoxin toxicity in this manner.

Q203. Answer: D

Explanation: Paroxysmal nocturnal dyspnea describes sudden nighttime episodes of breathlessness that awaken the patient from sleep. It occurs due to fluid redistribution from peripheral tissues to the lungs when lying flat. The patient typically needs to sit upright to relieve symptoms. Orthopnea refers to dyspnea occurring immediately upon lying down. Cheyne-Stokes respiration is a cyclic breathing pattern, and exertional dyspnea occurs during activity rather than at rest during sleep.

Q204. Answer: B

Explanation: ACE inhibitors reduce mortality in systolic heart failure by decreasing afterload and limiting maladaptive remodeling. They suppress the renin-angiotensin-aldosterone system, improving long-term outcomes. Loop diuretics relieve symptoms but do not reduce mortality. Calcium channel blockers are not routinely indicated in systolic heart failure. Nitrates may relieve symptoms but alone do not provide proven mortality benefit in this population.

Q205. Answer: A

Explanation: ST elevation in leads II, III, and aVF indicates an inferior myocardial infarction. The right coronary artery most commonly supplies the inferior wall of the heart. Occlusion leads to characteristic ECG findings in those leads. The left anterior descending artery typically causes anterior changes. The circumflex may cause lateral changes, and the diagonal branch supplies a smaller anterior-lateral region.

Q206. Answer: A

Explanation: Beck's triad includes hypotension, muffled heart sounds, and jugular venous distension. It is classic for cardiac tamponade due to pericardial fluid accumulation impairing ventricular filling. The reduced stroke volume leads to hypotension. Bounding pulses and widened pulse pressure are seen in conditions like aortic regurgitation. A loud S1 is more typical of mitral stenosis.

Q207. Answer: A

Explanation: Atrial fibrillation promotes blood stasis in the left atrium, especially in the left atrial appendage. This increases the risk of thrombus formation and systemic embolization. Stroke is the most feared complication. Pulmonary hypertension may coexist but is not the primary risk. Ventricular septal defects are structural abnormalities, and endocarditis requires infection, not merely arrhythmia.

Q208. Answer: B

Explanation: The S3 heart sound occurs during early diastole when blood rapidly fills a dilated ventricle. It is commonly associated with systolic heart failure and volume overload states. The sound reflects decreased ventricular compliance. S1 and S2 are normal heart sounds. S4 is associated with stiff ventricles and atrial contraction rather than rapid filling.

Q209. Answer: C

Explanation: An INR of 6.5 significantly increases bleeding risk. In the absence of bleeding, holding warfarin and monitoring is appropriate management. Dose adjustment may follow once INR returns to therapeutic range. Increasing warfarin would worsen coagulopathy. Thrombolytics and heparin would further increase bleeding risk and are not indicated in this situation.

Q210. Answer: B

Explanation: Aortic stenosis produces a harsh crescendo-decrescendo systolic murmur best heard at the right upper sternal border. Radiation to the carotid arteries is characteristic due to turbulent flow across the stenotic valve. Mitral regurgitation radiates toward the axilla. Pulmonary stenosis radiates toward the left shoulder. Tricuspid regurgitation increases with inspiration and is heard along the lower sternal border.

Q211. Answer: B

Explanation: Beta-blockers reduce heart rate and contractility, thereby decreasing myocardial oxygen demand. This helps relieve angina and reduces ischemic burden. They also prolong diastole, improving coronary perfusion. They do not directly cause coronary vasodilation. Increasing preload would worsen ischemia, and platelet aggregation is not enhanced by this drug class.

Q212. Answer: A

Explanation: CT pulmonary angiography is the diagnostic test of choice for suspected pulmonary embolism. It directly visualizes thrombi within pulmonary arteries. Immobilization increases venous thromboembolism risk. Echocardiography may show right heart strain but is not definitive. Stress testing and cardiac catheterization are not appropriate for suspected pulmonary embolism.

Q213. Answer: D

Explanation: Beta-blockers such as metoprolol are first-line agents for ventricular rate control in stable atrial fibrillation. They slow AV nodal conduction and reduce heart rate. Adenosine is used for supraventricular tachycardia. Atropine increases heart rate and is used for bradycardia. Epinephrine increases heart rate and contractility and is not used for rate control in atrial fibrillation.

Q214. Answer: B

Explanation: Aortic regurgitation leads to increased stroke volume and rapid diastolic runoff, creating a widened pulse pressure. This produces bounding peripheral pulses. Mitral stenosis typically causes normal or reduced pulse pressure. Cardiac tamponade results in narrowed pulse pressure. Pulmonary embolism does not characteristically cause widened pulse pressure.

Q215. Answer: C

Explanation: Myoglobin rises earliest after myocardial injury, often within 1-2 hours. However, it lacks specificity for cardiac muscle. Troponin is more specific and remains elevated longer. CK-MB rises slightly later than myoglobin. BNP is a marker of heart failure rather than acute myocardial infarction.

Q216. Answer: B

Explanation: Atropine increases heart rate by inhibiting vagal tone at the AV node. It is first-line therapy for symptomatic bradycardia with hypotension. Lidocaine and amiodarone treat ventricular arrhythmias. Magnesium sulfate is used in torsades de pointes and specific electrolyte disturbances.

Q217. Answer: C

Explanation: Smoking cessation significantly reduces cardiovascular morbidity and mortality. It improves endothelial function and decreases thrombosis risk. Even long-term smokers benefit substantially after quitting. Caffeine reduction and vitamins have minimal impact on cardiovascular risk. Increased protein intake does not directly reduce cardiovascular events.

Q218. Answer: C

Explanation: Pulseless electrical activity occurs when organized electrical activity is seen on the monitor but no mechanical cardiac output is present. It requires immediate resuscitation and identification of reversible causes. Ventricular fibrillation shows chaotic electrical activity. Asystole shows no electrical activity. Atrial flutter usually maintains some cardiac output.

Q219. Answer: B

Explanation: Positive blood cultures identifying a causative organism are a major diagnostic criterion for infective endocarditis. Persistent bacteremia supports the diagnosis when correlated with clinical findings. Elevated ESR is nonspecific. Tachycardia and chest pain are not diagnostic of this infection.

Q220. Answer: C

Explanation: Furosemide is a loop diuretic that reduces intravascular volume and decreases preload. It helps relieve pulmonary congestion in acute pulmonary edema. Dopamine may increase cardiac output but does not primarily reduce preload. Digoxin improves contractility but acts slowly. Warfarin is an anticoagulant and has no immediate effect on preload.

Q221. Answer: B

Explanation: Mitral stenosis produces a mid-diastolic rumbling murmur best heard at the cardiac apex. It is accentuated when the patient lies in the left lateral position due to closer proximity of the valve to the chest wall. Progressive dyspnea results from elevated left atrial pressures and pulmonary congestion. Aortic stenosis causes a systolic murmur, not diastolic. Mitral regurgitation produces a holosystolic murmur, and tricuspid stenosis is best heard at the lower sternal border.

Q222. Answer: B

Explanation: Left-sided heart failure leads to increased pressure in the pulmonary circulation. This causes fluid accumulation in the lungs, resulting in pulmonary congestion and dyspnea. Crackles and orthopnea are common findings. Peripheral edema and ascites are more typical of right-sided heart failure. Hepatomegaly also reflects systemic venous congestion rather than pulmonary involvement.

Q223. Answer: C

Explanation: Amiodarone is commonly used for the treatment of stable ventricular tachycardia. It works by prolonging repolarization and decreasing automaticity. It is effective in both atrial and ventricular arrhythmias. Adenosine is used for supraventricular tachycardia. Atropine treats bradycardia, and verapamil is primarily used for supraventricular rhythms rather than ventricular tachycardia.

Q224. Answer: C

Explanation: Acute pericarditis causes sharp, pleuritic chest pain that worsens when lying flat and improves when sitting up or leaning forward. This positional component is characteristic. Stable angina is typically exertional and relieved by rest. Pulmonary embolism presents with dyspnea and pleuritic pain but not usually positional relief. Myocardial infarction pain is persistent and not relieved by position change.

Q225. Answer: D

Explanation: B-type natriuretic peptide is released from ventricular myocardium in response to volume overload and increased wall stretch. Elevated levels support the diagnosis of heart failure exacerbation. Troponin indicates myocardial injury rather than volume overload. Creatinine assesses renal function, and hemoglobin evaluates anemia. BNP specifically correlates with ventricular pressure and volume changes.

Q226. Answer: A

Explanation: Hypertrophic cardiomyopathy predisposes patients to malignant ventricular arrhythmias. Sudden cardiac death is a significant risk, especially in younger individuals and athletes. The abnormal myocardial architecture increases electrical instability. Aortic dissection is not a primary complication. Pulmonary fibrosis is unrelated, and while endocarditis can occur, it is not the predominant risk.

Q227. Answer: B

Explanation: Ventricular fibrillation is a shockable rhythm requiring immediate unsynchronized defibrillation. Early defibrillation improves survival by restoring organized electrical activity. Atropine is used for bradycardia. Synchronized cardioversion is reserved for unstable tachyarrhythmias with a pulse. Adenosine treats supraventricular tachycardia.

Q228. Answer: A

Explanation: Deep vein thrombosis commonly presents with unilateral swelling, pain, and warmth. It poses a significant risk for pulmonary embolism if untreated. Early recognition and anticoagulation are critical. Cellulitis involves infection and skin changes. Peripheral artery disease causes claudication rather than swelling. Lymphedema is typically chronic and non-painful.

Q229. Answer: A

Explanation: Right-sided heart failure leads to systemic venous congestion. Jugular venous distension reflects elevated right atrial pressure. Peripheral edema and hepatomegaly are also common. Crackles and orthopnea are signs of left-sided failure. An S3 at the apex is typically associated with left ventricular dysfunction.

Q230. Answer: C

Explanation: Clopidogrel inhibits the P2Y12 ADP receptor on platelets, reducing platelet aggregation. It is commonly used in acute coronary syndrome and after stent placement. Aspirin inhibits cyclooxygenase and thromboxane production. Heparin enhances antithrombin activity. Warfarin inhibits vitamin K-dependent clotting factors.

Q231. Answer: D

Explanation: Severe aortic stenosis limits cardiac output during exertion. This can result in syncope due to inadequate cerebral perfusion. Exertional chest pain and dyspnea are also common. Hemoptysis is more associated with pulmonary pathology. Polyuria is unrelated, and cyanosis at birth indicates congenital heart disease.

Q232. Answer: D

Explanation: ST elevation in contiguous leads indicates transmural myocardial injury. It is a hallmark of ST-elevation myocardial infarction. Rapid recognition allows timely reperfusion therapy. Sinus tachycardia is nonspecific. AV block and premature atrial contractions may occur but are not specific indicators of infarction.

Q233. Answer: A

Explanation: Sildenafil enhances nitric oxide-mediated vasodilation. Combined use with nitrates can cause profound hypotension. This interaction may lead to syncope or shock. Beta-blockers, ACE inhibitors, and statins can be safely combined with nitrates under medical supervision.

Q234. Answer: B

Explanation: Activated partial thromboplastin time monitors therapeutic levels of unfractionated heparin. It reflects intrinsic pathway activity and guides dose adjustments. INR monitors warfarin therapy. Platelet count is monitored for heparin-induced thrombocytopenia. D-dimer assesses clot breakdown rather than heparin effect.

Q235. Answer: A

Explanation: Diffuse ST elevation with PR depression is characteristic of acute pericarditis. The changes are widespread rather than confined to a coronary distribution. PR depression reflects atrial involvement. STEMI shows localized ST elevation with reciprocal changes. Unstable angina does not produce ST elevation, and aortic aneurysm does not cause this ECG pattern.

Q236. Answer: B

Explanation: An S4 occurs due to atrial contraction against a stiff, noncompliant ventricle. Ventricular hypertrophy decreases compliance and produces this sound. It is heard just before S1. Dilated cardiomyopathy more often produces S3. Acute mitral regurgitation causes a systolic murmur, and atrial septal defect has characteristic fixed splitting of S2.

Q237. Answer: A

Explanation: Elevated low-density lipoprotein contributes to plaque formation in arterial walls. It promotes cholesterol deposition and inflammation. Lowering LDL reduces cardiovascular events. High HDL is protective. Low triglycerides and low total cholesterol are not associated with increased atherosclerotic risk.

Q238. Answer: A

Explanation: Epinephrine is the primary treatment for anaphylaxis. It increases vascular tone, improves blood pressure, and relieves bronchospasm. Prompt administration prevents cardiovascular collapse. Antihistamines and steroids are adjunctive therapies. Albuterol treats bronchospasm but does not correct hypotension.

Q239. Answer: A

Explanation: Chronic hypertension increases afterload on the left ventricle. This leads to concentric left ventricular hypertrophy as the myocardium thickens to compensate. Over time, this may result in diastolic dysfunction. Right atrial enlargement is secondary to pulmonary disease. Septal defects and patent ductus arteriosus are congenital conditions.

Q240. Answer: D

Explanation: Early beta-blocker therapy reduces myocardial oxygen demand and decreases arrhythmia risk after myocardial infarction. It improves survival and limits infarct size. Routine long-term oxygen is not indicated unless hypoxia is present. Prolonged bed rest increases complications. Prophylactic antiarrhythmics have not demonstrated survival benefit and may increase risk.

Q241. Answer: C

Explanation: Hypotension with clear lungs and elevated jugular venous pressure suggests right ventricular infarction. The right ventricle fails to pump blood effectively to the pulmonary circulation, leading to systemic venous congestion. Lung fields remain clear because left ventricular function may be preserved. Papillary muscle rupture typically causes pulmonary edema. Ventricular septal rupture leads to a harsh murmur and heart failure signs.

Q242. Answer: A

Explanation: Sublingual nitroglycerin rapidly dilates coronary arteries and reduces preload. This decreases myocardial oxygen demand and relieves angina pain. It acts quickly when placed under the tongue. Digoxin improves contractility but does not provide immediate pain relief. Furosemide reduces fluid overload, and atorvastatin lowers cholesterol over time.

Q243. Answer: D

Explanation: Vegetations on infected heart valves can dislodge and embolize. When emboli travel to cerebral circulation, they may cause stroke. Systemic embolization is a serious complication of infective endocarditis. Pulmonary fibrosis and chronic bronchitis are unrelated respiratory conditions. Peptic ulcer disease is not a direct consequence of endocarditis.

Q244. Answer: A

Explanation: Reduced cardiac output reflects impaired pumping ability of the left ventricle. Systolic dysfunction leads to decreased forward flow and systemic hypoperfusion. Ejection fraction would decline rather than increase. BNP levels typically rise with worsening heart failure. Pulse pressure changes are not as specific as direct reduction in output.

Q245. Answer: D

Explanation: Patent ductus arteriosus produces a continuous machinery-like murmur due to persistent flow between the aorta and pulmonary artery. The murmur spans systole and diastole. This occurs because the ductus fails to close after birth. Atrial and ventricular septal defects usually produce systolic murmurs. Mitral valve prolapse produces a mid-systolic click with murmur.

Q246. Answer: A

Explanation: Lisinopril, an ACE inhibitor, increases bradykinin levels. Accumulation of bradykinin can cause a persistent dry cough. This side effect is common and may necessitate switching to an angiotensin receptor blocker. Losartan does not typically cause cough. Amlodipine and metoprolol are not associated with this symptom.

Q247. Answer: A

Explanation: Mitral regurgitation allows blood to flow back into the left atrium during systole. Chronic volume overload leads to left atrial enlargement. This may predispose to atrial fibrillation. Right-sided structures enlarge secondary to pulmonary hypertension, not directly from mitral regurgitation. The pulmonary artery itself does not enlarge as a primary chamber response.

Q248. Answer: C

Explanation: Atrial fibrillation produces chaotic atrial electrical activity. This results in absence of organized P waves and irregularly irregular ventricular response. It is the most common sustained arrhythmia. Atrial flutter has sawtooth flutter waves. Ventricular tachycardia is typically regular and wide complex. Sinus arrhythmia maintains normal P waves.

Q249. Answer: D

Explanation: Pulsus paradoxus is an exaggerated drop in systolic blood pressure during inspiration. It is commonly seen in cardiac tamponade due to impaired ventricular filling. The phenomenon reflects ventricular interdependence. Hypertension and hyperlipidemia do not cause this sign. Aortic stenosis does not typically produce pulsus paradoxus.

Q250. Answer: B

Explanation: Beta-blockers reduce sympathetic overactivation in heart failure. They improve ventricular remodeling and decrease mortality. Long-term therapy improves survival and reduces hospitalization. Thiazide diuretics relieve mild fluid retention but do not reduce mortality. Calcium channel blockers are not routinely beneficial in reduced ejection fraction. Nitrates alone do not confer survival benefit.

Q251. Answer: D

Explanation: Central line placement carries risk of pneumothorax, particularly with subclavian access. Sudden dyspnea and chest pain after the procedure suggest lung collapse. Decreased breath sounds may be noted on the affected side. Pericarditis and endocarditis are not immediate complications. Myocardial infarction would present differently and is less directly related.

Q252. Answer: D

Explanation: Troponin I is highly specific for cardiac muscle injury. It remains elevated for several days after myocardial infarction. This specificity makes it the preferred diagnostic marker. CK-MB is less specific. Myoglobin rises early but lacks cardiac specificity. LDH is nonspecific and less commonly used.

Q253. Answer: C

Explanation: Hypertensive emergency involves severe blood pressure elevation with evidence of target organ damage. Headache and visual changes suggest neurologic involvement. Immediate blood pressure reduction is required. Hypertensive urgency lacks acute organ damage. White coat hypertension is situational. Orthostatic hypotension is low blood pressure upon standing.

Q254. Answer: A

Explanation: Renal artery stenosis decreases renal perfusion. This activates the renin-angiiotensin-aldosterone system, leading to hypertension. It is a common cause of secondary hypertension. Essential hypertension is primary without identifiable cause. Hyperlipidemia and sedentary lifestyle contribute to cardiovascular risk but do not directly cause secondary hypertension.

Q255. Answer: D

Explanation: Early ambulation promotes venous return and reduces stasis. This lowers the risk of clot formation in immobilized patients. Mechanical prophylaxis and anticoagulation may also be used. Strict bed rest increases thrombotic risk. Fluid restriction and dietary fat intake do not directly prevent thrombosis.

Q256. Answer: D

Explanation: Atrial flutter produces characteristic sawtooth flutter waves on ECG. These are most prominent in the inferior leads. Ventricular response may be regular or variable. Irregular baseline without P waves describes atrial fibrillation. Wide QRS complexes suggest ventricular rhythm. Prolonged PR interval indicates first-degree AV block.

Q257. Answer: C

Explanation: Statins inhibit HMG-CoA reductase and reduce hepatic cholesterol synthesis. They significantly lower LDL levels and reduce cardiovascular events. They are first-line therapy for dyslipidemia. Niacin and fibrates primarily affect triglycerides and HDL. Digoxin has no lipid-lowering properties.

Q258. Answer: B

Explanation: Intermittent claudication presents as leg pain during exertion relieved by rest. It results from reduced arterial blood flow to muscles. Peripheral arterial disease is caused by atherosclerosis. Leg swelling is more typical of venous disease. Cyanosis at birth indicates congenital defects, and productive cough is respiratory.

Q259. Answer: A

Explanation: Troponin remains elevated for up to 7-10 days after myocardial infarction. This prolonged elevation assists in late diagnosis. Myoglobin rises and falls quickly. CK-MB returns to baseline within a few days. AST is nonspecific and less commonly used.

Q260. Answer: D

Explanation: Mitral stenosis results in obstruction of blood flow from the left atrium to the left ventricle. This causes elevated left atrial pressure and pulmonary congestion. The valve opening is narrowed, restricting diastolic filling. Mitral regurgitation involves backward flow rather than obstruction. Aortic and tricuspid regurgitation affect different valves and mechanisms.

Q261. Answer: C

Explanation: Chronic atrial fibrillation promotes clot formation in the left atrium due to blood stasis. These clots can embolize to cerebral circulation and cause an ischemic stroke. Sudden focal neurological deficits strongly suggest embolic origin in this context. Intracranial hemorrhage is possible but less directly associated with atrial fibrillation. Hypoglycemia can cause altered mental status but not focal deficits of this type. Migraine aura does not typically cause persistent motor weakness.

Q262. Answer: C

Explanation: Pink frothy sputum and diffuse crackles indicate acute pulmonary edema. Rapid diuresis with an intravenous loop diuretic reduces preload and pulmonary congestion. Prompt treatment improves oxygenation and decreases respiratory distress. Supine positioning worsens pulmonary fluid accumulation. Rapid IV fluids and oral hydration would exacerbate volume overload.

Q263. Answer: D

Explanation: Beta-blockers decrease heart rate and contractility, lowering myocardial oxygen demand. This helps control ischemic chest pain in unstable angina. They also reduce arrhythmia risk. Epinephrine and dopamine increase heart rate and oxygen demand. Atropine increases heart rate and would worsen ischemia.

Q264. Answer: A

Explanation: Severe back pain and hypotension after femoral access suggest retroperitoneal bleeding. This complication can occur if the arterial puncture site is above the inguinal ligament. Blood accumulates in the retroperitoneal space and may not be externally visible. Pulmonary embolism presents with dyspnea and chest pain. Pericarditis and aortic stenosis are unrelated to catheterization site complications.

Q265. Answer: C

Explanation: Rapid weight gain in heart failure indicates fluid retention. Increasing dyspnea suggests worsening volume overload. Prompt adjustment of diuretic therapy can prevent hospitalization. Sodium intake should be restricted rather than increased. Beta-blockers should not be discontinued abruptly unless directed. Reassurance alone is insufficient in this scenario.

Q266. Answer: D

Explanation: A significant platelet drop during heparin therapy suggests heparin-induced thrombocytopenia. This immune-mediated reaction increases thrombotic risk. Immediate discontinuation of heparin is necessary to prevent complications. Continuing or increasing the dose worsens risk. Aspirin does not treat the underlying immune response.

Q267. Answer: B

Explanation: Inferior myocardial infarction often involves the right coronary artery, which supplies the AV node. This may result in bradycardia. Atropine increases heart rate by blocking vagal tone. Lidocaine and amiodarone treat ventricular arrhythmias. Nitroglycerin may worsen hypotension in this situation.

Q268. Answer: B

Explanation: Mechanical heart valves increase risk of thromboembolism. Long-term anticoagulation with warfarin is necessary to prevent clot formation. INR monitoring ensures therapeutic levels. Aspirin alone is insufficient. Clopidogrel and digoxin do not provide adequate anticoagulation for mechanical valves.

Q269. Answer: D

Explanation: Tearing chest pain with widened mediastinum suggests aortic dissection. CT angiography is the preferred imaging modality for rapid diagnosis. Early detection is critical for surgical planning. Stress testing is contraindicated. Holter monitoring is used for arrhythmias. Echocardiography may help but CT provides definitive imaging.

Q270. Answer: A

Explanation: Long-acting nitrates reduce frequency of angina episodes by decreasing preload and myocardial oxygen demand. They are used for prophylaxis rather than acute relief. Short-acting nitrates treat acute episodes only. Thrombolytics are used in acute myocardial infarction. Epinephrine increases cardiac workload and is not appropriate.

Q271. Answer: C

Explanation: Rapid blood pressure reduction can decrease cerebral perfusion. This may cause confusion or altered mental status. Gradual lowering is recommended in most hypertensive emergencies. Reflex hypertension does not cause hypotension. Hyperglycemia and fluid overload are not direct consequences of rapid antihypertensive therapy.

Q272. Answer: D

Explanation: Echocardiography assesses chamber size and ejection fraction. It provides detailed evaluation of ventricular function. Dilated cardiomyopathy is characterized by enlarged ventricles and reduced contractility. Chest X-ray shows cardiac silhouette but not function. ECG shows electrical activity. D-dimer assesses thrombosis.

Q273. Answer: D

Explanation: Sudden severe headache during thrombolytic therapy may indicate intracranial hemorrhage. Immediate discontinuation of the infusion is necessary. Rapid evaluation is critical to prevent further bleeding. Continuing therapy increases risk. Aspirin would worsen bleeding. Ambulation is inappropriate.

Q274. Answer: D

Explanation: Rest pain relieved by dependent positioning indicates severe arterial insufficiency. Dangling the legs increases gravitational blood flow. This is a sign of advanced peripheral arterial disease. Venous insufficiency causes swelling and aching. Normal aging and muscle strain do not produce this pattern.

Q275. Answer: A

Explanation: ST elevation in leads V1-V4 indicates anterior wall myocardial infarction. These leads correspond to the anterior portion of the left ventricle. The left anterior descending artery commonly supplies this region. Inferior changes appear in II, III, and aVF. Lateral changes appear in I, aVL, V5, and V6.

Q276. Answer: D

Explanation: Spironolactone is a potassium-sparing diuretic. It can cause potassium retention leading to hyperkalemia. Monitoring serum potassium is essential to prevent arrhythmias. Hypokalemia is more common with loop diuretics. Hyponatremia and hypercalcemia are less directly associated with this medication.

Q277. Answer: B

Explanation: Severe symptomatic aortic stenosis requires valve replacement. Surgical or transcatheter intervention relieves obstruction and improves survival. Medical therapy alone does not correct the mechanical obstruction. Lifestyle changes and medications may provide temporary symptom relief but are not definitive.

Q278. Answer: A

Explanation: Prolonged immobility increases risk of deep vein thrombosis. Clot migration to pulmonary arteries results in pulmonary embolism. Sudden dyspnea and pleuritic chest pain are classic symptoms. Myocarditis develops more gradually. Stable angina is exertional. Pericardial effusion presents differently with muffled heart sounds.

Q279. Answer: B

Explanation: Chronic hyperglycemia damages vascular endothelium. It accelerates atherosclerosis and increases cardiovascular risk. Combined with hypertension, it significantly raises morbidity. Caffeine intake and mild dehydration have minimal impact on long-term cardiovascular disease progression. Seasonal allergies are unrelated to atherosclerosis.

Q280. Answer: B

Explanation: Cardiac rehabilitation improves functional capacity and promotes lifestyle modification. It reduces risk of recurrent cardiovascular events. Structured exercise and education enhance recovery and adherence. It does not cure coronary disease. Medications and follow-up remain essential components of care.

Q281. Answer: D

Explanation: Preserved ejection fraction with symptoms of heart failure suggests diastolic dysfunction. Long-standing hypertension leads to left ventricular hypertrophy and reduced compliance. An S4 heart sound reflects atrial contraction against a stiff ventricle. Systolic heart failure would demonstrate reduced ejection fraction. Myocarditis and right ventricular infarction present differently and are not characterized by chronic preserved function.

Q282. Answer: D

Explanation: Hypotension and bradycardia are known adverse effects of intravenous amiodarone. Temporarily stopping the infusion prevents further hemodynamic compromise. Continuous monitoring is essential during administration. Increasing the rate would worsen instability. Ambulation is unsafe in hypotension. Potassium administration is not indicated unless a documented deficiency exists.

Q283. Answer: C

Explanation: Muffled heart sounds, jugular venous distension, and hypotension represent classic findings of cardiac tamponade. Trauma may cause pericardial bleeding leading to compression of the heart. This restricts ventricular filling and decreases cardiac output. Tension pneumothorax causes absent breath sounds. Myocardial contusion presents with arrhythmias. Pulmonary edema produces crackles rather than distended neck veins.

Q284. Answer: B

Explanation: Atrial fibrillation predisposes to systemic embolization. An embolus to mesenteric arteries can cause acute mesenteric ischemia. Sudden severe abdominal pain out of proportion to examination findings is characteristic. Peptic ulcer and appendicitis have different clinical courses. Pancreatitis is associated with elevated pancreatic enzymes and risk factors such as gallstones or alcohol use.

Q285. Answer: B

Explanation: Sodium promotes water retention through osmotic mechanisms. In heart failure, excess fluid worsens congestion and edema. Restricting sodium helps control volume overload. It does not directly prevent arrhythmias. Heart rate and oxygen saturation are not primarily affected by sodium intake.

Q286. Answer: A

Explanation: Pale, cool extremity with weak pulses suggests compromised arterial blood flow. Acute limb ischemia is a vascular emergency requiring prompt intervention. Delayed treatment may result in tissue necrosis. Cellulitis presents with warmth and redness. Venous thrombosis typically causes swelling and warmth. Lymphedema develops gradually and is not acutely limb-threatening.

Q287. Answer: C

Explanation: Hemodynamic instability with atrial fibrillation requires immediate synchronized cardioversion. Low blood pressure indicates poor cardiac output. Electrical cardioversion restores sinus rhythm quickly. Oral medications act too slowly in unstable patients. Observation alone is unsafe, and aspirin does not correct arrhythmia.

Q288. Answer: C

Explanation: Statins may cause myopathy or rhabdomyolysis. Elevated creatine kinase indicates muscle injury. Early detection prevents severe complications. Potassium levels may change in rhabdomyolysis but are not primary screening tests. Hemoglobin and D-dimer are unrelated to statin-induced muscle injury.

Q289. Answer: C

Explanation: Stable angina occurs with predictable exertion and resolves with rest. It reflects fixed coronary artery obstruction. Symptoms are reproducible under similar activity levels. Unstable angina is unpredictable and may occur at rest. Variant angina involves coronary vasospasm. Myocardial infarction causes prolonged, persistent pain.

Q290. Answer: A

Explanation: Left ventricular failure reduces systemic perfusion. Decreased cardiac output limits blood flow to the brain and kidneys. This results in confusion and oliguria. Increased cerebral perfusion would not cause confusion. Hypervolemia contributes to congestion but not directly to decreased urine output. Pulmonary hypertension primarily affects right heart function.

Q291. Answer: A

Explanation: A positive D-dimer suggests possible thrombosis but is not definitive. Compression venous ultrasound confirms presence of clot. Imaging guides appropriate anticoagulation therapy. Thrombolytics are reserved for severe cases. Stress testing and aspirin are not diagnostic for deep vein thrombosis.

Q292. Answer: B

Explanation: Hypertrophic cardiomyopathy increases risk of malignant ventricular arrhythmias. Sudden collapse during exertion is often due to ventricular tachycardia or fibrillation. Myocardial disarray creates electrical instability. Pulmonary embolism and dehydration are possible but less directly linked. Hypoglycemia causes gradual symptoms rather than sudden cardiac arrest.

Q293. Answer: C

Explanation: ACE inhibitors can cause angioedema due to bradykinin accumulation. Facial swelling and airway compromise are life-threatening. Immediate discontinuation and airway management are required. Dry cough is common but not life-threatening. Electrolyte disturbances do not cause facial swelling.

Q294. Answer: D

Explanation: Chronic venous insufficiency leads to pooling of blood in lower extremities. Red blood cells leak into tissues and break down, depositing hemosiderin. This causes brown discoloration. Arterial blockage results in pale skin. Cyanosis causes bluish color. Acute thrombosis presents with swelling and pain rather than pigmentation changes.

Q295. Answer: C

Explanation: Ventricular septal rupture after myocardial infarction causes a new holosystolic murmur. Blood shunts between ventricles, leading to pulmonary congestion. This is a mechanical complication requiring urgent intervention. Aortic dissection presents with tearing chest pain. Pericarditis produces positional chest pain. Stable angina does not cause acute murmur.

Q296. Answer: A

Explanation: An INR of 9 significantly increases bleeding risk. Vitamin K reverses excessive anticoagulation. It helps restore clotting factor production. Increasing warfarin or adding heparin would worsen bleeding. Permanent discontinuation depends on indication and is not automatically required.

Q297. Answer: D

Explanation: An implantable cardioverter-defibrillator detects and terminates life-threatening arrhythmias. It reduces risk of sudden cardiac death in high-risk patients. It does not directly improve ventricular function. Blood pressure control and medications remain necessary. The device is protective rather than curative.

Q298. Answer: B

Explanation: Echocardiography visualizes vegetations on heart valves. It is essential for diagnosing infective endocarditis. Transesophageal imaging provides detailed assessment. Chest X-ray and ECG offer supportive information but do not confirm vegetations. Lipid profile is unrelated.

Q299. Answer: A

Explanation: Diabetes causes both neuropathy and accelerated atherosclerosis. Numbness reflects nerve damage, while diminished pulses indicate arterial disease. Combined complications increase risk of ulcers and amputation. Myocarditis and pericardial effusion involve cardiac inflammation. Atrial septal defect is congenital.

Q300. Answer: D

Explanation: Sudden respiratory compromise after surgery requires immediate lung assessment. Auscultation helps identify pneumothorax, atelectasis, or fluid accumulation. Early recognition guides rapid intervention. Surgical dressing assessment is important but secondary. Bowel sounds and anthropometric measurements are not priorities in acute respiratory distress.

Question (301-400)

Q301. Why does left ventricular hypertrophy initially develop in response to chronic hypertension?
(A) To decrease myocardial oxygen consumption
(B) To compensate for increased afterload
(C) To reduce preload
(D) To improve coronary perfusion

Q302. What is the primary physiological reason beta-blockers reduce mortality after myocardial infarction?
(A) They increase myocardial contractility
(B) They reduce sympathetic stimulation
(C) They directly dilate coronary arteries
(D) They dissolve coronary thrombi

Q303. Why does mitral stenosis lead to pulmonary hypertension over time?
(A) Increased right ventricular contractility
(B) Reduced systemic vascular resistance
(C) Backward transmission of elevated left atrial pressure
(D) Increased aortic pressure

Q304. What is the conceptual difference between preload and afterload?
(A) Preload reflects end-diastolic stretch; afterload reflects resistance to ejection
(B) Preload occurs during systole; afterload occurs during diastole
(C) Preload is heart rate dependent; afterload is oxygen dependent
(D) Preload is ventricular resistance; afterload is ventricular volume

Q305. Why does atrial fibrillation increase the risk of thromboembolism?
(A) Turbulent blood flow in coronary arteries
(B) Blood stasis in the atria
(C) Increased ventricular contraction
(D) Enhanced platelet production

Q306. Why is troponin considered more specific than CK-MB for myocardial infarction?
(A) It is unaffected by renal function
(B) It remains elevated longer and is cardiac-specific
(C) It detects skeletal muscle injury
(D) It rises earlier

Q307. Why does severe aortic stenosis cause exertional syncope?
(A) Increased pulmonary pressure
(B) Excessive preload
(C) Elevated heart rate at rest
(D) Reduced cerebral perfusion during increased demand

Q308. What is the rationale for sodium restriction in heart failure management?
(A) To decrease fluid retention and preload
(B) To stimulate aldosterone release
(C) To increase renal perfusion
(D) To prevent arrhythmias directly

Q309. Why does right-sided heart failure commonly lead to peripheral edema?
(A) Elevated systemic venous pressure
(B) Reduced left atrial pressure
(C) Increased pulmonary artery pressure
(D) Decreased coronary perfusion

Q310. Why are ACE inhibitors beneficial in slowing progression of heart failure?
(A) They increase heart rate
(B) They suppress renin-angiotensin-aldosterone activation
(C) They enhance platelet aggregation
(D) They directly repair myocardium

Q311. What is the underlying cause of S3 heart sound in systolic heart failure?
(A) Rapid ventricular filling into a dilated chamber
(B) Atrial contraction against stiff ventricle
(C) Turbulent systolic ejection
(D) Closure of semilunar valves

Q312. Why does pulmonary embolism lead to sudden hypoxia?
(A) Increased hemoglobin concentration
(B) Enhanced oxygen diffusion
(C) Obstruction of pulmonary blood flow
(D) Reduced alveolar ventilation only

Q313. Why is anticoagulation required in patients with mechanical heart valves?
(A) To reduce ventricular hypertrophy
(B) To prevent infection
(C) To increase cardiac output
(D) To prevent thrombus formation on artificial surfaces

Q314. What is the physiological effect of nitrates in angina management?

(A) Increase myocardial oxygen demand
(B) Dilate veins and reduce preload
(C) Increase systemic vascular resistance
(D) Stimulate sympathetic activity

Q315. Why does chronic diabetes accelerate atherosclerosis?
(A) Increased insulin sensitivity
(B) Lower LDL levels
(C) Reduced platelet adhesion
(D) Endothelial damage from persistent hyperglycemia

Q316. What is the conceptual reason hypertrophic cardiomyopathy increases risk of sudden cardiac death?
(A) Increased hemoglobin
(B) Elevated preload
(C) Reduced coronary blood flow only
(D) Electrical instability from myocardial disarray

Q317. Why does cardiac tamponade cause hypotension?
(A) Reduced systemic resistance
(B) Restricted ventricular filling
(C) Excess sympathetic output
(D) Increased stroke volume

Q318. What is the purpose of synchronized cardioversion in unstable tachyarrhythmias?
(A) Increase automaticity
(B) Deliver shock during T wave
(C) Deliver shock synchronized with R wave
(D) Stimulate vagal tone

Q319. Why does chronic venous insufficiency lead to skin ulceration?
(A) Persistent venous hypertension
(B) Arterial occlusion
(C) Reduced platelet count
(D) Acute embolism

Q320. Why is early ambulation recommended after surgery to prevent thromboembolism?
(A) Increase platelet aggregation
(B) Elevate blood pressure
(C) Decrease oxygen demand
(D) Reduce venous stasis

Q321. A 64-year-old male with a history of smoking presents with crushing chest pain radiating to his left arm for 45 minutes. ECG shows ST elevation in leads II, III, and aVF. Blood pressure is 90/60 mmHg and heart rate is 52 bpm. What is the most appropriate immediate intervention?
(A) Encourage ambulation
(B) Administer IV atropine
(C) Administer sublingual nitroglycerin
(D) Start high-dose beta-blocker

Q322. A 70-year-old woman with heart failure reports waking at night gasping for air. She has bilateral crackles and elevated BNP levels. What is the underlying mechanism of her symptoms?
(A) Fluid redistribution to lungs when supine
(B) Increased hemoglobin levels
(C) Coronary vasospasm
(D) Reduced preload

Q323. A patient with atrial fibrillation is scheduled for cardioversion. The rhythm has been present for 5 days. What is the priority concern before the procedure?
(A) Hyperlipidemia
(B) Electrolyte imbalance
(C) Hypertension
(D) Presence of atrial thrombus

Q324. A postoperative patient suddenly develops shortness of breath, tachycardia, and pleuritic chest pain on day three after hip surgery. What is the most likely diagnosis?
(A) Pulmonary embolism
(B) Pneumonia
(C) Atelectasis
(D) Myocardial infarction

Q325. A 59-year-old male with uncontrolled hypertension complains of tearing chest pain radiating to the back. Blood pressures differ between arms. What is the priority diagnostic test?
(A) Holter monitor
(B) CT angiography
(C) Lipid panel
(D) Exercise stress test

Q326. A patient with chronic venous insufficiency presents with a shallow ulcer near the medial ankle. The surrounding skin is brownish and edematous. What is the most appropriate initial management?
(A) Compression therapy
(B) Surgical bypass
(C) High-dose anticoagulation

(D) Immediate amputation

Q327. A patient receiving thrombolytic therapy for STEMI develops sudden weakness on one side and difficulty speaking. What complication should be suspected?

(A) Cardiogenic shock
(B) Pulmonary edema
(C) Reinfarction
(D) Intracranial hemorrhage

Q328. A 66-year-old woman with diabetes presents with atypical symptoms including nausea, fatigue, and mild shortness of breath. ECG shows ST depression. What is the most likely diagnosis?

(A) Panic attack
(B) Gastroenteritis
(C) Stable angina
(D) Non-ST elevation myocardial infarction

Q329. A patient with severe aortic stenosis becomes dizzy while climbing stairs. What is the physiological explanation?

(A) Fixed obstruction limiting cardiac output
(B) Elevated hemoglobin
(C) Excess coronary vasodilation
(D) Increased preload

Q330. A patient with right-sided heart failure presents with abdominal distension and liver enlargement. What is the primary cause?

(A) Mitral valve stenosis
(B) Coronary artery blockage
(C) Pulmonary congestion
(D) Systemic venous congestion

Q331. A patient with long-term uncontrolled hyperlipidemia presents with calf pain when walking that resolves with rest. What is the underlying condition?

(A) Deep vein thrombosis
(B) Sciatic nerve compression
(C) Chronic venous insufficiency
(D) Peripheral arterial disease

Q332. A patient with dilated cardiomyopathy reports worsening fatigue and palpitations. ECG reveals frequent premature ventricular contractions. What is the main risk?

(A) Stroke
(B) Aortic rupture
(C) Pulmonary infection
(D) Ventricular tachyarrhythmia

Q333. A 74-year-old patient with hypertension develops sudden severe headache and blood pressure of 230/120 mmHg with blurred vision. What is the most appropriate management approach?

(A) Oral medication and discharge
(B) Observation only
(C) Rapid normalization of BP within minutes
(D) Gradual controlled reduction with IV medication

Q334. A patient with mitral regurgitation complains of increasing fatigue and shortness of breath. Echocardiogram shows left atrial enlargement. What complication is most likely to develop?

(A) Pericarditis
(B) Atrial fibrillation
(C) Ventricular septal defect
(D) Pulmonary embolism

Q335. A patient with acute pulmonary edema is placed on high-flow oxygen but remains hypoxic. What is the next priority intervention?

(A) Initiate noninvasive positive pressure ventilation
(B) Provide oral hydration
(C) Increase IV fluids
(D) Encourage deep breathing exercises

Q336. A patient undergoing hemodialysis experiences chest pain and hypotension during treatment. What is the likely cause?

(A) Hyperglycemia
(B) Rapid fluid removal causing decreased preload
(C) Fluid overload
(D) Increased hemoglobin

Q337. A 60-year-old patient presents with fever, chills, and a new systolic murmur after dental work. What is the most likely diagnosis?

(A) Rheumatic fever
(B) Myocardial infarction
(C) Pericardial effusion
(D) Infective endocarditis

Q338. A patient with chronic heart failure suddenly develops rapid weight gain and decreased urine output. What does this indicate?

(A) Improved cardiac output

(B) Renal stone formation
(C) Fluid retention
(D) Dehydration

Q339. A patient with known coronary artery disease experiences chest pain at rest lasting 20 minutes. ECG shows no ST elevation. What is the likely diagnosis?
(A) Stable angina
(B) Aortic stenosis
(C) Pericarditis
(D) Unstable angina

Q340. A patient with left ventricular failure is prescribed an ACE inhibitor. After several weeks, blood pressure improves and symptoms decrease. What is the primary therapeutic effect responsible?
(A) Decreased coronary perfusion
(B) Reduced afterload and remodeling
(C) Increased heart rate
(D) Increased sodium retention

Q341. A 67-year-old man with a history of anterior myocardial infarction presents with sudden onset of severe shortness of breath and a new loud systolic murmur. Blood pressure is dropping rapidly. What is the most likely complication?
(A) Stable angina
(B) Chronic mitral stenosis
(C) Ventricular septal rupture
(D) Pulmonary fibrosis

Q342. A patient with long-standing atrial fibrillation stops taking anticoagulation therapy. Two weeks later, he develops sudden vision loss in one eye. What is the most likely cause?
(A) Embolic event
(B) Retinal detachment
(C) Cataract progression
(D) Glaucoma

Q343. A 58-year-old woman with poorly controlled diabetes presents with chest discomfort and shortness of breath. ECG is nondiagnostic, but troponin is elevated. What is the most likely diagnosis?
(A) Stable angina
(B) Pericarditis
(C) Panic disorder
(D) NSTEMI

Q344. A patient with chronic hypertension suddenly develops severe chest pain radiating to the jaw and diaphoresis. ECG shows ST elevation in V2-V5. What artery is most likely occluded?
(A) Posterior descending artery
(B) Right coronary artery
(C) Left anterior descending artery
(D) Left circumflex artery

Q345. A patient recovering from cardiac surgery develops low blood pressure, rising central venous pressure, and muffled heart sounds. What is the immediate priority?
(A) Evaluate for pericardial tamponade
(B) Administer diuretics
(C) Encourage ambulation
(D) Increase IV fluids

Q346. A 73-year-old patient with peripheral arterial disease presents with a cold, pulseless leg and severe pain at rest. What is the most appropriate immediate action?
(A) Apply compression stockings
(B) Initiate emergency vascular evaluation
(C) Elevate the limb
(D) Encourage walking

Q347. A patient with acute myocardial infarction develops cardiogenic shock. Blood pressure is 75/40 mmHg and urine output is minimal. What is the primary cause?
(A) Peripheral vasodilation
(B) Severe pump failure
(C) Hypervolemia
(D) Excess preload

Q348. A patient with mitral valve prolapse experiences palpitations and anxiety. What is the underlying structural issue?
(A) Valve calcification
(B) Aortic narrowing
(C) Leaflet displacement into left atrium
(D) Ventricular septal defect

Q349. A hospitalized patient receiving IV fluids rapidly develops crackles and dyspnea. What is the most likely cause?
(A) Fluid overload
(B) Asthma attack
(C) Pulmonary embolism
(D) Hypoglycemia

Q350. A 62-year-old man with long-standing smoking history presents with progressive leg pain and diminished femoral pulses. What is the likely diagnosis?
(A) Peripheral arterial disease
(B) Deep vein thrombosis
(C) Chronic venous insufficiency
(D) Cellulitis
Q351. A patient with uncontrolled hypertension presents with sudden onset confusion and weakness. CT scan reveals intracerebral hemorrhage. What is the primary contributing factor?
(A) Dehydration
(B) Low cholesterol levels
(C) Excess preload
(D) Chronic vascular wall stress
Q352. A patient with severe heart failure is started on spironolactone and later develops peaked T waves on ECG. What electrolyte imbalance is suspected?
(A) Hypokalemia
(B) Hypocalcemia
(C) Hyponatremia
(D) Hyperkalemia
Q353. A patient experiences chest pain relieved by nitroglycerin but recurring more frequently at rest. What does this pattern suggest?
(A) Stable angina
(B) Gastroesophageal reflux
(C) Unstable angina
(D) Improved angina
Q354. A patient undergoing dialysis complains of chest pain and hypotension near the end of treatment. What is the most likely reason?
(A) Rapid decrease in circulating volume
(B) Excess fluid retention
(C) Elevated potassium
(D) Increased afterload
Q355. A patient with long-standing mitral stenosis develops hemoptysis and worsening dyspnea. What is the most likely progression?
(A) Pulmonary hypertension
(B) Acute myocardial infarction
(C) Aortic rupture
(D) Ventricular septal defect
Q356. A patient presents with syncope and ECG shows complete heart block. What is the definitive treatment?
(A) Oral beta-blocker
(B) Diuretic therapy
(C) Permanent pacemaker
(D) Aspirin therapy
Q357. A patient with coronary artery disease reports chest pain during emotional stress. What is the physiological trigger?
(A) Reduced heart rate
(B) Increased myocardial oxygen demand
(C) Decreased sympathetic tone
(D) Elevated hemoglobin
Q358. A patient with chronic heart failure develops worsening edema and ascites despite medication compliance. What is the likely explanation?
(A) Improved cardiac output
(B) Disease progression
(C) Increased exercise
(D) Excess sodium restriction
Q359. A patient with infective endocarditis suddenly develops flank pain and hematuria. What complication should be suspected?
(A) Kidney stone
(B) Urinary tract infection
(C) Dehydration
(D) Renal embolism
Q360. A patient with severe coronary artery disease undergoes successful angioplasty with stent placement. What is the primary purpose of dual antiplatelet therapy afterward?
(A) Reduce preload
(B) Prevent stent thrombosis
(C) Increase hemoglobin
(D) Prevent infection
Q361. A 69-year-old woman with a history of heart failure presents with increasing shortness of breath, orthopnea, and bilateral leg swelling. On examination, she has an S3 gallop and crackles at both lung bases. What is the most likely cause of her worsening symptoms?
(A) Progressive left ventricular dysfunction
(B) Acute pulmonary embolism
(C) Acute asthma exacerbation
(D) Dehydration

Q362. A 75-year-old patient with atrial fibrillation presents with sudden onset severe leg pain, pallor, and absence of distal pulses. What is the most likely diagnosis?
(A) Chronic venous insufficiency
(B) Deep vein thrombosis
(C) Acute arterial embolism
(D) Peripheral neuropathy
Q363. A patient with hypertrophic cardiomyopathy experiences chest pain during exertion despite normal coronary arteries. What explains this symptom?
(A) Coronary artery blockage
(B) Increased myocardial oxygen demand from thickened muscle
(C) Pulmonary hypertension
(D) Reduced hemoglobin
Q364. A 63-year-old patient develops sudden hypotension and tachycardia after a large anterior myocardial infarction. Lungs are clear and jugular veins are distended. What is the most likely cause?
(A) Papillary muscle rupture
(B) Left ventricular failure
(C) Right ventricular infarction
(D) Ventricular septal defect
Q365. A patient on long-term warfarin therapy presents with severe headache and INR of 8.5. What is the most concerning complication?
(A) Myocardial infarction
(B) Intracranial hemorrhage
(C) Deep vein thrombosis
(D) Ischemic stroke
Q366. A patient with severe aortic stenosis reports worsening fatigue and dyspnea on minimal exertion. Echocardiography shows reduced ejection fraction. What does this indicate?
(A) Improved cardiac output
(B) Resolution of obstruction
(C) Disease progression with ventricular failure
(D) Compensated disease
Q367. A patient admitted for unstable angina suddenly develops ST elevation and crushing chest pain. What does this change signify?
(A) Panic attack
(B) Development of STEMI
(C) Gastroesophageal reflux
(D) Resolution of ischemia
Q368. A patient with chronic heart failure is noncompliant with medications and presents with rapid weight gain and severe dyspnea. What is the primary pathophysiological process?
(A) Fluid overload due to neurohormonal activation
(B) Increased cardiac contractility
(C) Decreased aldosterone
(D) Reduced sympathetic activity
Q369. A patient with infective endocarditis develops sudden chest pain and shortness of breath. CT scan reveals pulmonary emboli. What is the likely source?
(A) Coronary plaque rupture
(B) Left-sided vegetation
(C) Right-sided vegetation
(D) Aortic dissection
Q370. A patient with peripheral arterial disease presents with a non-healing ulcer on the toes. The foot is cool and hairless. What is the underlying cause?
(A) Acute infection
(B) Venous hypertension
(C) Lymphatic obstruction
(D) Arterial insufficiency
Q371. A 72-year-old patient with heart failure presents with confusion and low urine output. Blood pressure is 85/50 mmHg. What is the primary mechanism?
(A) Pulmonary vasodilation
(B) Elevated hemoglobin
(C) Hypervolemia
(D) Decreased cardiac output
Q372. A patient with atrial fibrillation and rapid ventricular response complains of dizziness and palpitations. Blood pressure is 88/60 mmHg. What is the next step?
(A) Synchronized cardioversion
(B) Observation only
(C) Lifestyle counseling
(D) Oral anticoagulation
Q373. A patient receiving ACE inhibitors develops persistent dry cough. What is the physiological reason?
(A) Bradykinin accumulation
(B) Increased aldosterone

(C) Sodium retention
(D) Elevated hemoglobin

Q374. A patient with long-standing mitral regurgitation develops atrial fibrillation. What structural change predisposed to this arrhythmia?
(A) Left atrial enlargement
(B) Right ventricular hypertrophy
(C) Pulmonary valve stenosis
(D) Aortic dilation

Q375. A patient hospitalized for myocardial infarction suddenly becomes unresponsive with no palpable pulse. Monitor shows chaotic irregular waves. What is the immediate intervention?
(A) Synchronized cardioversion
(B) Atropine injection
(C) Oral beta-blocker
(D) Defibrillation

Q376. A patient with severe heart failure reports abdominal swelling and early satiety. What is the likely cause?
(A) Acute gastritis
(B) Peptic ulcer disease
(C) Pulmonary edema
(D) Ascites from systemic congestion

Q377. A patient presents with chest pain that worsens with deep inspiration and improves when sitting forward. ECG shows diffuse ST elevation. What is the diagnosis?
(A) Acute pericarditis
(B) Aortic stenosis
(C) STEMI
(D) Stable angina

Q378. A patient with uncontrolled hypertension develops left ventricular hypertrophy. What is the primary long-term risk?
(A) Decreased oxygen demand
(B) Improved compliance
(C) Reduced blood pressure
(D) Diastolic dysfunction

Q379. A patient with coronary artery disease experiences chest pain during emotional stress. What mediates this response?
(A) Parasympathetic activation
(B) Sympathetic stimulation increasing oxygen demand
(C) Reduced heart rate
(D) Increased venous return only

Q380. A patient with advanced heart failure is evaluated for implantable cardioverter-defibrillator placement. What is the primary goal of this device?
(A) Cure coronary artery disease
(B) Increase ejection fraction
(C) Eliminate medication need
(D) Prevent fatal arrhythmias

Q381. A 68-year-old man with a history of inferior myocardial infarction develops sudden hypotension, clear lung sounds, and elevated jugular venous pressure. What is the most appropriate immediate management?
(A) Provide rapid intravenous fluid bolus
(B) Administer intravenous nitroglycerin
(C) Initiate morphine therapy
(D) Start high-dose diuretics

Q382. A 72-year-old patient with chronic atrial fibrillation presents with worsening fatigue and dyspnea. Echocardiogram shows reduced left ventricular function. What is the likely mechanism?
(A) Acute pulmonary embolism
(B) Pericardial tamponade
(C) Persistent tachycardia leading to cardiomyopathy
(D) Mitral valve stenosis

Q383. A patient with severe coronary artery disease suddenly develops tearing chest pain radiating to the back. Blood pressure is markedly elevated. What life-threatening condition must be ruled out immediately?
(A) Aortic dissection
(B) Pericarditis
(C) Unstable angina
(D) Pulmonary edema

Q384. A patient with chronic heart failure presents with worsening lower extremity edema and hepatomegaly. Which pathophysiological process explains these findings?
(A) Increased systemic venous pressure
(B) Increased hemoglobin production
(C) Decreased preload
(D) Reduced pulmonary vascular resistance

Q385. A patient experiences syncope during exertion. Examination reveals a harsh systolic murmur radiating to the carotids. What is the most likely diagnosis?
(A) Tricuspid regurgitation
(B) Mitral regurgitation
(C) Aortic stenosis
(D) Pulmonary embolism
Q386. A hospitalized patient with myocardial infarction develops sudden shortness of breath and pink frothy sputum. What is the immediate complication?
(A) Pericarditis
(B) Right ventricular infarction
(C) Deep vein thrombosis
(D) Pulmonary edema
Q387. A patient with infective endocarditis complains of sudden weakness in one arm and difficulty speaking. What is the most likely cause?
(A) Anxiety attack
(B) Septic embolic stroke
(C) Migraine
(D) Hypoglycemia
Q388. A 65-year-old patient with long-standing hypertension develops left ventricular hypertrophy. What compensatory change initially occurs in the myocardium?
(A) Chamber dilation
(B) Decreased muscle mass
(C) Valve calcification
(D) Wall thickening to reduce wall stress
Q389. A patient with peripheral arterial disease reports rest pain in the feet, especially at night. What does this indicate?
(A) Venous congestion
(B) Neuropathic pain only
(C) Critical limb ischemia
(D) Improved perfusion
Q390. A patient receiving beta-blocker therapy for heart failure develops bradycardia and dizziness. What is the mechanism of action responsible?
(A) Increased sympathetic activity
(B) Vasoconstriction
(C) Reduced heart rate and myocardial oxygen demand
(D) Sodium retention
Q391. A patient with mitral stenosis presents with hemoptysis and worsening dyspnea. What is the underlying pathophysiology?
(A) Decreased left atrial pressure
(B) Increased systemic vascular resistance
(C) Pulmonary venous hypertension
(D) Coronary occlusion
Q392. A patient with acute coronary syndrome develops new onset confusion and hypotension. What is the likely explanation?
(A) Anxiety
(B) Pulmonary embolism
(C) Cardiogenic shock causing cerebral hypoperfusion
(D) Hyperglycemia
Q393. A patient with atrial fibrillation complains of palpitations and shortness of breath. ECG shows irregularly irregular rhythm. What is the main hemodynamic consequence?
(A) Loss of atrial kick reducing ventricular filling
(B) Increased stroke volume
(C) Increased coronary perfusion
(D) Reduced afterload
Q394. A patient presents with chest pain that improves when leaning forward and worsens when lying flat. What physical finding is most consistent?
(A) Pericardial friction rub
(B) Absent pulses
(C) Systolic murmur at apex
(D) Carotid bruit
Q395. A patient with chronic heart failure has persistent hyponatremia. What is the most likely cause?
(A) Increased renal perfusion
(B) Hyperkalemia
(C) Decreased aldosterone secretion
(D) Excessive water retention due to neurohormonal activation
Q396. A patient with coronary artery disease experiences sudden cardiac arrest. Monitor reveals ventricular tachycardia without pulse. What is the immediate intervention?
(A) Oral antiarrhythmic medication
(B) Defibrillation
(C) Intravenous fluids only
(D) Observation

Q397. A patient with uncontrolled hypertension develops retinal hemorrhages and papilledema. What condition does this indicate?

(A) Hypertensive emergency
(B) Chronic anemia
(C) Glaucoma
(D) Stable hypertension

Q398. A patient with severe dilated cardiomyopathy presents with fatigue and low blood pressure. What is the primary structural abnormality?

(A) Enlarged ventricular chamber with reduced contractility
(B) Narrowed aortic valve
(C) Thickened ventricular wall
(D) Normal chamber size

Q399. A patient recovering from myocardial infarction suddenly develops a new holosystolic murmur at the apex and acute pulmonary edema. What is the likely cause?

(A) Chronic bronchitis
(B) Stable angina
(C) Aortic dissection
(D) Papillary muscle rupture

Q400. A patient with advanced heart failure is placed on a low-sodium diet. What is the primary goal of this intervention?

(A) Increase blood pressure
(B) Enhance myocardial contractility
(C) Increase cardiac output
(D) Reduce fluid retention and preload

Answer Key and Explanation (301-400)

Q301. Answer: B

Explanation: Chronic hypertension increases systemic vascular resistance, creating elevated afterload against which the left ventricle must pump. To maintain cardiac output, myocardial fibers thicken, leading to concentric hypertrophy. This structural adaptation initially preserves systolic function. Over time, the thickened ventricle becomes stiff and less compliant. The long-term consequence is diastolic dysfunction and eventual heart failure progression.

Q302. Answer: B

Explanation: After myocardial infarction, excessive sympathetic activation increases heart rate and oxygen demand. Beta-blockers blunt this response by blocking adrenergic receptors. This decreases myocardial workload and reduces risk of fatal arrhythmias. Lower oxygen demand limits infarct expansion. The overall effect improves survival and reduces recurrent events.

Q303. Answer: C

Explanation: Mitral stenosis restricts blood flow from the left atrium to the left ventricle. This causes left atrial pressure to rise chronically. Elevated pressure is transmitted backward into pulmonary veins and capillaries. Persistent pulmonary venous congestion leads to vascular remodeling and pulmonary hypertension. Eventually, right ventricular strain may develop as a secondary consequence.

Q304. Answer: A

Explanation: Preload refers to the degree of myocardial fiber stretch at end-diastole, determined by venous return. It represents the filling pressure of the ventricle before contraction. Afterload represents the resistance the ventricle must overcome to eject blood. Increased systemic vascular resistance elevates afterload. Both factors significantly influence stroke volume and cardiac performance.

Q305. Answer: B

Explanation: Atrial fibrillation causes ineffective atrial contraction and chaotic electrical activity. This leads to pooling and stasis of blood, especially in the left atrial appendage. Stagnant blood promotes thrombus formation. If dislodged, clots can embolize to systemic circulation. Stroke is a common and serious consequence of this mechanism.

Q306. Answer: B

Explanation: Troponin proteins are highly specific to cardiac muscle tissue. Their elevation indicates myocardial cell injury with greater accuracy than CK-MB. Troponin remains elevated for several days, aiding late diagnosis. CK-MB can also rise with skeletal muscle damage. The specificity of troponin makes it the preferred biomarker for infarction confirmation.

Q307. Answer: D

Explanation: Aortic stenosis obstructs left ventricular outflow. During exertion, systemic vasodilation occurs but cardiac output cannot increase adequately. This leads to reduced cerebral perfusion and syncope. The fixed obstruction limits the ability to meet metabolic demand. Over time, the condition may progress to heart failure if untreated.

Q308. Answer: A

Explanation: Sodium intake promotes water retention through osmotic mechanisms. In heart failure, excess volume worsens ventricular filling pressures and pulmonary congestion. Restricting sodium helps reduce preload and fluid accumulation. This supports symptom control and reduces hospitalization risk. It complements pharmacologic therapy such as diuretics.

Q309. Answer: A

Explanation: Right-sided heart failure impairs forward flow into the pulmonary circulation. Blood backs up into systemic venous circulation. Elevated venous pressure forces fluid into interstitial tissues. Dependent areas such as legs and ankles are most affected. Chronic congestion may also cause hepatomegaly and ascites.

Q310. Answer: B

Explanation: ACE inhibitors block conversion of angiotensin I to angiotensin II. This reduces vasoconstriction and aldosterone-mediated fluid retention. By decreasing afterload and preload, ventricular workload is reduced. They also limit maladaptive remodeling of the myocardium. These mechanisms collectively slow disease progression and improve survival.

Q311. Answer: A

Explanation: S3 occurs during early diastole when blood rapidly fills a dilated ventricle. In systolic heart failure, ventricular dilation reduces compliance. The sudden deceleration of blood produces the characteristic sound. It is often associated with volume overload. Presence of S3 in adults usually indicates pathological ventricular dysfunction.

Q312. Answer: C

Explanation: Pulmonary embolism blocks blood flow in pulmonary arteries. This creates ventilation-perfusion mismatch, where ventilated alveoli receive inadequate perfusion. Oxygen exchange becomes inefficient. The result is acute hypoxemia and dyspnea. Severity depends on clot size and location within pulmonary circulation.

Q313. Answer: D

Explanation: Mechanical valves are thrombogenic due to artificial surfaces. Blood contact with prosthetic material promotes clot formation. Anticoagulation reduces risk of systemic embolization. Without therapy, stroke and valve obstruction may occur. Lifelong management is typically necessary to maintain therapeutic levels.

Q314. Answer: B

Explanation: Nitrates primarily dilate venous capacitance vessels. This reduces venous return and decreases preload. Lower ventricular filling pressure reduces myocardial wall stress. Consequently, oxygen demand declines and angina symptoms improve. Coronary vasodilation may also contribute to relief.

Q315. Answer: D

Explanation: Persistent hyperglycemia damages vascular endothelium. This promotes inflammation and lipid deposition in arterial walls. Glycation of proteins further contributes to plaque formation. Diabetic patients have increased risk of premature coronary artery disease. Aggressive glycemic control reduces vascular complications.

Q316. Answer: D

Explanation: Hypertrophic cardiomyopathy involves abnormal myocardial fiber arrangement. This structural disorganization creates electrical instability. Ventricular arrhythmias may occur unpredictably. Sudden cardiac death often results from ventricular fibrillation. Risk stratification is essential in affected individuals.

Q317. Answer: B

Explanation: In cardiac tamponade, fluid accumulation in the pericardial sac compresses the heart. Ventricular filling during diastole is restricted. Reduced filling leads to decreased stroke volume. Cardiac output falls, resulting in hypotension. Prompt drainage is required to restore hemodynamic stability.

Q318. Answer: C

Explanation: Synchronized cardioversion times the shock with the R wave. This avoids delivering energy during ventricular repolarization. Delivering a shock during the vulnerable period could trigger ventricular fibrillation. The procedure restores organized electrical activity. It is indicated in unstable patients with a pulse.

Q319. Answer: A

Explanation: Chronic venous hypertension impairs capillary circulation. Fluid and proteins leak into surrounding tissues. Poor oxygen and nutrient delivery damages skin integrity. Over time, ulcers develop, typically around the medial malleolus. Management focuses on improving venous return and compression therapy.

Q320. Answer: D

Explanation: Immobility promotes venous pooling in lower extremities. Stasis increases risk of clot formation. Early ambulation enhances calf muscle pump activity. Improved venous return reduces thromboembolic risk. This intervention complements pharmacologic prophylaxis when indicated.

Q321. Answer: B

Explanation: ST elevation in inferior leads suggests inferior myocardial infarction, often involving the right coronary artery. Bradycardia and hypotension indicate possible AV nodal involvement. Atropine increases heart rate and improves cardiac output in symptomatic bradycardia. Nitroglycerin may worsen hypotension in inferior infarction. Beta-blockers are contraindicated in unstable hypotension. Ambulation is unsafe during acute infarction.

Q322. Answer: A

Explanation: Paroxysmal nocturnal dyspnea occurs when lying flat causes fluid from peripheral tissues to shift into pulmonary circulation. In heart failure, the left ventricle cannot manage the increased volume. This leads to pulmonary congestion and acute breathlessness. Elevated BNP supports volume overload. The condition reflects worsening left ventricular dysfunction.

Q323. Answer: D

Explanation: Atrial fibrillation lasting more than 48 hours increases risk of thrombus formation in the left atrium. Cardioversion can dislodge a clot, causing stroke. Anticoagulation or transesophageal echocardiography is required beforehand. Electrolytes are important but secondary to embolic risk. Hypertension and hyperlipidemia do not pose immediate procedural threats.

Q324. Answer: A

Explanation: Recent orthopedic surgery increases risk of deep vein thrombosis. Sudden dyspnea and pleuritic chest pain suggest embolization to pulmonary arteries. Tachycardia is a common finding. Pneumonia develops more gradually with fever and productive cough. Atelectasis causes mild dyspnea but not sudden severe symptoms.

Q325. Answer: B

Explanation: Tearing chest pain with unequal arm blood pressures strongly suggests aortic dissection. CT angiography provides rapid visualization of the aorta. Early diagnosis is essential for surgical management. Stress testing is contraindicated in acute chest pain. Holter monitoring and lipid panels are not useful in emergencies.

Q326. Answer: A

Explanation: Venous ulcers result from chronic venous hypertension and poor return. Compression therapy improves venous return and reduces edema. It promotes healing and prevents recurrence. Surgical bypass is used for arterial disease. Anticoagulation is not indicated unless thrombosis exists. Amputation is not first-line treatment.

Q327. Answer: D

Explanation: Thrombolytics increase bleeding risk, including intracranial hemorrhage. Sudden neurological deficits suggest cerebral bleeding. Immediate discontinuation and urgent imaging are required. Reinfarction presents with recurrent chest pain. Cardiogenic shock causes hypotension. Pulmonary edema presents with respiratory distress.

Q328. Answer: D

Explanation: Diabetic patients often present with atypical myocardial infarction symptoms. ST depression indicates subendocardial ischemia. Elevated cardiac biomarkers would confirm NSTEMI. Gastroenteritis does not cause ECG changes. Stable angina resolves with rest. Panic attacks do not produce ischemic ECG findings.

Q329. Answer: A

Explanation: Severe aortic stenosis creates a fixed outflow obstruction. During exertion, the heart cannot increase output to meet demand. Systemic vasodilation reduces cerebral perfusion. This leads to exertional dizziness or syncope. The underlying problem is mechanical obstruction at the valve.

Q330. Answer: D

Explanation: Right-sided heart failure impairs forward blood flow into pulmonary circulation. Blood backs up into systemic veins. Elevated venous pressure leads to hepatomegaly and ascites. Pulmonary congestion is typical of left-sided failure. Coronary blockage causes ischemia, not systemic congestion.

Q331. Answer: D

Explanation: Calf pain triggered by exertion and relieved by rest describes intermittent claudication. It is caused by atherosclerotic narrowing of peripheral arteries. Hyperlipidemia accelerates plaque formation. Deep vein thrombosis causes persistent pain and swelling. Venous insufficiency leads to edema rather than exertional pain.

Q332. Answer: D

Explanation: Dilated cardiomyopathy predisposes to electrical instability. Frequent premature ventricular contractions may degenerate into sustained ventricular arrhythmias. These arrhythmias can lead to sudden cardiac death. Stroke risk is more associated with atrial fibrillation. Pulmonary infection and aortic rupture are not direct consequences.

Q333. Answer: D

Explanation: Severe hypertension with neurologic symptoms indicates hypertensive emergency. Controlled blood pressure reduction with IV agents prevents further organ damage. Rapid normalization may compromise cerebral perfusion. Oral medication alone is insufficient. Close monitoring in a critical setting is required.

Q334. Answer: B

Explanation: Chronic mitral regurgitation causes volume overload of the left atrium. Enlargement predisposes to atrial fibrillation. Irregular rhythm further reduces cardiac efficiency. Pulmonary embolism is unrelated to valve regurgitation directly. Pericarditis and septal defects are different pathological processes.

Q335. Answer: A

Explanation: Noninvasive positive pressure ventilation improves oxygenation by reducing preload and enhancing alveolar recruitment. It decreases work of breathing in pulmonary edema. Increasing fluids worsens congestion. Oral hydration and simple breathing exercises are insufficient in acute respiratory distress. Prompt ventilatory support improves outcomes.

Q336. Answer: B

Explanation: Excessive ultrafiltration during dialysis reduces intravascular volume. Decreased preload lowers cardiac output. This may cause hypotension and chest discomfort. Careful fluid management is necessary. Fluid overload would increase blood pressure, not decrease it.

Q337. Answer: D

Explanation: Dental procedures can introduce bacteria into the bloodstream. Bacteremia may seed heart valves, causing infective endocarditis. Fever and new murmur are classic findings. Prompt blood cultures and echocardiography are required. Rheumatic fever is less common in older adults.

Q338. Answer: C

Explanation: Rapid weight gain in heart failure indicates fluid accumulation. Decreased urine output suggests worsening renal perfusion and congestion. Early recognition allows medication adjustment. Improved cardiac output would increase urine production. Dehydration would cause weight loss.

Q339. Answer: D

Explanation: Chest pain at rest suggests unstable angina. It reflects plaque rupture and partial thrombosis. Absence of ST elevation differentiates it from STEMI. Stable angina occurs predictably with exertion. Prompt evaluation is necessary to prevent progression to infarction.

Q340. Answer: B

Explanation: ACE inhibitors decrease angiotensin II production. This reduces systemic vascular resistance and afterload. They also limit ventricular remodeling and progression of heart failure. The combined effects improve symptoms and survival. They do not increase sodium retention or heart rate.

Q341. Answer: C

Explanation: A new loud systolic murmur with acute heart failure after myocardial infarction suggests a mechanical complication. Ventricular septal rupture creates a left-to-right shunt, leading to pulmonary congestion and hypotension. This condition is life-threatening and requires urgent surgical intervention. Stable angina does not produce new murmurs. Chronic mitral stenosis develops gradually and does not present acutely after infarction.

Q342. Answer: A

Explanation: Discontinuation of anticoagulation in atrial fibrillation increases thrombus risk. Emboli may travel to retinal arteries, causing sudden painless vision loss. This represents systemic embolization from the left atrium. Retinal detachment often causes flashes and floaters. Glaucoma and cataracts typically cause gradual visual changes.

Q343. Answer: D

Explanation: Elevated troponin indicates myocardial injury. In the absence of ST elevation, this presentation is consistent with non-ST elevation myocardial infarction. Diabetic patients often have atypical symptoms. Stable angina does not elevate cardiac biomarkers. Pericarditis typically presents with diffuse ST elevation and positional pain.

Q344. Answer: C

Explanation: ST elevation in anterior leads V2-V5 indicates anterior wall myocardial infarction. The left anterior descending artery supplies this region. Occlusion causes significant myocardial damage and high mortality risk. Prompt reperfusion therapy is essential. Inferior wall infarctions involve different leads and arteries.

Q345. Answer: A

Explanation: Hypotension with elevated venous pressure and muffled heart sounds suggests cardiac tamponade. Postoperative bleeding may accumulate in the pericardial sac. Urgent evaluation and possible pericardiocentesis are required. Diuretics would worsen hypotension. Increasing fluids alone does not relieve compression.

Q346. Answer: B

Explanation: A cold, pulseless limb indicates acute arterial occlusion. Immediate vascular intervention is required to prevent tissue loss. Delays may result in necrosis and amputation. Compression stockings are contraindicated in arterial insufficiency. Elevation worsens perfusion.

Q347. Answer: B

Explanation: Cardiogenic shock occurs when the heart fails to pump effectively. Extensive myocardial damage reduces cardiac output. Hypotension and decreased organ perfusion follow. Urine output declines due to reduced renal blood flow. Peripheral vasodilation is not the primary mechanism in cardiogenic shock.

Q348. Answer: C

Explanation: Mitral valve prolapse involves bulging of valve leaflets into the left atrium during systole. This may cause regurgitation and palpitations. It is often benign but can produce symptoms. Valve calcification is characteristic of stenosis. Septal defects and aortic narrowing involve different structures.

Q349. Answer: A

Explanation: Rapid infusion of fluids may exceed cardiac capacity, especially in vulnerable patients. Excess volume increases pulmonary capillary pressure. Fluid leaks into alveoli, causing pulmonary edema. Crackles and dyspnea are classic findings. Asthma involves bronchospasm, not fluid accumulation.

Q350. Answer: A

Explanation: Smoking accelerates atherosclerosis in peripheral arteries. Diminished pulses and exertional leg pain suggest arterial obstruction. Peripheral arterial disease reduces blood supply to lower extremities. Deep vein thrombosis causes swelling and warmth. Venous insufficiency causes edema and pigmentation changes rather than pulse reduction.

Q351. Answer: D

Explanation: Chronic hypertension weakens cerebral vessel walls. Persistent pressure leads to microaneurysm formation and rupture. Intracerebral hemorrhage is a severe complication. Low cholesterol and dehydration are not primary causes. Managing blood pressure reduces recurrence risk.

Q352. Answer: D

Explanation: Spironolactone is a potassium-sparing diuretic. Elevated potassium levels may occur, leading to ECG changes such as peaked T waves. Severe hyperkalemia can cause life-threatening arrhythmias. Monitoring serum potassium is essential during therapy.

Q353. Answer: C

Explanation: Increasing frequency of chest pain occurring at rest indicates unstable angina. It suggests plaque instability and higher risk of infarction. Prompt evaluation and treatment are necessary. Stable angina remains predictable. Nitroglycerin relieves ischemic pain but does not eliminate underlying risk.

Q354. Answer: A

Explanation: Rapid fluid removal during dialysis reduces circulating blood volume. Decreased preload lowers cardiac output and blood pressure. This may cause chest discomfort.

Careful adjustment of ultrafiltration rates helps prevent this complication.

Q355. Answer: A

Explanation: Chronic elevation of left atrial pressure in mitral stenosis leads to pulmonary venous congestion. Over time, this causes pulmonary hypertension. Hemoptysis may occur from ruptured bronchial veins. Progressive dyspnea reflects worsening pulmonary vascular changes.

Q356. Answer: C

Explanation: Complete heart block results in loss of atrioventricular conduction. Ventricular escape rhythms are often inadequate. A permanent pacemaker restores coordinated electrical activity. Medication alone is insufficient. Timely pacing prevents recurrent syncope and sudden death.

Q357. Answer: B

Explanation: Emotional stress activates the sympathetic nervous system. Increased heart rate and blood pressure raise myocardial oxygen demand. In the presence of coronary narrowing, supply cannot meet demand. Ischemia and chest pain result. Stress management is part of comprehensive care.

Q358. Answer: B

Explanation: Heart failure is a progressive condition. Despite adherence, ventricular function may deteriorate. Fluid accumulation reflects worsening pump function. Medication adjustment or advanced therapy may be required. Increased exercise or sodium restriction would not cause worsening edema.

Q359. Answer: D

Explanation: Vegetations from infected valves may embolize systemically. Renal artery embolism can cause flank pain and hematuria. Prompt imaging is required to confirm diagnosis. Kidney stones present with colicky pain but are unrelated to endocarditis.

Q360. Answer: B

Explanation: Stent placement injures vascular endothelium and exposes thrombogenic surfaces. Platelet activation may lead to acute stent thrombosis. Dual antiplatelet therapy reduces this risk. Adherence is critical to prevent life-threatening complications.

Q361. Answer: A

Explanation: The presence of orthopnea, S3 gallop, and pulmonary crackles indicates worsening left ventricular systolic dysfunction. Progressive pump failure leads to elevated left-sided filling pressures. Fluid accumulates in the lungs, producing dyspnea and crackles. Peripheral edema may occur as the condition advances. Pulmonary embolism presents more abruptly and asthma does not cause S3 gallop.

Q362. Answer: C

Explanation: Sudden severe pain, pallor, and pulselessness indicate acute arterial occlusion. Atrial fibrillation predisposes to thrombus formation in the atrium. Embolization to peripheral arteries can cause limb ischemia. This condition requires immediate vascular intervention. Deep vein thrombosis typically presents with swelling and warmth, not pallor and pulselessness.

Q363. Answer: B

Explanation: In hypertrophic cardiomyopathy, the thickened ventricular wall increases oxygen demand. Microvascular dysfunction may also impair perfusion. Even without coronary artery disease, ischemia can occur. Exertion further increases demand, leading to chest pain. The problem is structural hypertrophy rather than epicardial artery obstruction.

Q364. Answer: C

Explanation: Clear lung fields with hypotension and elevated jugular venous pressure suggest right ventricular infarction. The right ventricle fails to pump blood effectively to the lungs. This results in systemic venous congestion without pulmonary edema. Anterior infarctions may extend to involve the right ventricle in some cases.

Q365. Answer: B

Explanation: An INR of 8.5 indicates excessive anticoagulation. Severe headache raises concern for intracranial bleeding. Warfarin increases risk of hemorrhagic complications when supratherapeutic. Immediate reversal and imaging are necessary. Ischemic stroke is less likely with elevated INR.

Q366. Answer: C

Explanation: Severe aortic stenosis initially causes concentric hypertrophy with preserved function. Over time, chronic pressure overload leads to ventricular failure and reduced ejection fraction. Worsening symptoms indicate decompensation. Surgical intervention is often required at this stage.

Q367. Answer: B

Explanation: ST elevation with persistent chest pain indicates progression to ST-elevation myocardial infarction. This reflects complete coronary artery occlusion. Immediate reperfusion therapy is required. Unstable angina may progress if untreated. The ECG change confirms transmural ischemia.

Q368. Answer: A

Explanation: Heart failure activates renin-angiotensin-aldosterone and sympathetic systems. This promotes sodium and water retention. Noncompliance worsens volume overload. Rapid weight gain reflects fluid accumulation. Increased filling pressures cause dyspnea and edema.

Q369. Answer: C

Explanation: Right-sided infective endocarditis commonly affects the tricuspid valve. Vegetations may embolize to the pulmonary circulation. This results in septic pulmonary emboli. Left-sided vegetations embolize to systemic circulation instead.

Q370. Answer: D

Explanation: Peripheral arterial disease reduces blood flow to distal tissues. Poor perfusion impairs wound healing. Cool temperature and hair loss indicate chronic arterial insufficiency. Ulcers typically occur on toes or pressure points. Restoring circulation is essential for healing.

Q371. Answer: D

Explanation: Hypotension in heart failure reflects inadequate pump function. Reduced cardiac output decreases cerebral and renal perfusion. This causes confusion and oliguria. The underlying issue is systemic hypoperfusion. Immediate stabilization is required to prevent organ failure.

Q372. Answer: A

Explanation: Hemodynamic instability in atrial fibrillation requires urgent cardioversion. Hypotension and dizziness indicate compromised cardiac output. Electrical cardioversion restores organized rhythm quickly. Delaying intervention increases risk of deterioration.

Q373. Answer: A

Explanation: ACE inhibitors prevent breakdown of bradykinin. Elevated bradykinin irritates airway mucosa. This leads to a persistent dry cough. The effect is benign but bothersome. Switching to an angiotensin receptor blocker may relieve symptoms.

Q374. Answer: A

Explanation: Chronic mitral regurgitation increases volume load in the left atrium. Enlargement disrupts normal conduction pathways. This structural remodeling predisposes to atrial fibrillation. The arrhythmia further impairs cardiac efficiency.

Q375. Answer: D

Explanation: Chaotic irregular waves without pulse indicate ventricular fibrillation. Immediate defibrillation is required. Early shock increases survival by restoring organized rhythm. Delayed treatment decreases success rates.

Q376. Answer: D

Explanation: Right-sided heart failure causes systemic venous congestion. Fluid accumulates in the abdominal cavity, producing ascites. Abdominal distension and early satiety result from pressure on stomach. This reflects advanced disease progression.

Q377. Answer: A

Explanation: Positional chest pain with diffuse ST elevation is characteristic of acute pericarditis. Inflammation of the pericardium causes sharp pleuritic pain. Sitting forward reduces pericardial irritation. Unlike STEMI, ST elevation is widespread rather than localized.

Q378. Answer: D

Explanation: Left ventricular hypertrophy reduces ventricular compliance. Stiff myocardium impairs diastolic filling. This leads to diastolic heart failure over time. Chronic pressure overload drives this maladaptive remodeling.

Q379. Answer: B

Explanation: Emotional stress triggers sympathetic activation. Heart rate and blood pressure rise. Increased myocardial oxygen demand exceeds supply in narrowed coronary arteries. Ischemia and chest pain result. Stress management is part of prevention strategy.

Q380. Answer: D

Explanation: Implantable cardioverter-defibrillators detect and terminate life-threatening ventricular arrhythmias. They reduce risk of sudden cardiac death. The device does not reverse structural heart disease. Medications and lifestyle modifications remain essential components of care.

Q381. Answer: A

Explanation: Hypotension with elevated jugular venous pressure and clear lungs suggests right ventricular infarction. The right ventricle depends on adequate preload to maintain cardiac output. Administering fluids increases preload and improves hemodynamic stability. Vasodilators and diuretics would reduce preload and worsen hypotension. Prompt recognition prevents progression to cardiogenic shock.

Q382. Answer: C

Explanation: Chronic uncontrolled rapid ventricular response can cause tachycardia-induced cardiomyopathy. Sustained high heart rates impair ventricular filling and contractility. Over time, this leads to reduced ejection fraction. Controlling rate or restoring rhythm can improve function. The mechanism is functional deterioration from persistent tachyarrhythmia.

Q383. Answer: A

Explanation: Tearing chest pain radiating to the back is classic for aortic dissection. Severe hypertension is a major risk factor. Immediate imaging is required because delay can be fatal. The pain quality differs from typical ischemic chest pain. Rapid diagnosis guides urgent surgical or medical management.

Q384. Answer: A

Explanation: Right-sided heart failure causes blood to back up into systemic veins. Elevated venous pressure leads to peripheral edema and liver congestion. Hepatomegaly results from chronic passive congestion. The problem stems from impaired forward flow on the right side. Managing volume status is essential to relieve symptoms.

Q385. Answer: C

Explanation: Exertional syncope with a systolic murmur radiating to the carotids is characteristic of aortic stenosis. The narrowed valve restricts blood flow during activity. Cardiac output cannot increase appropriately, causing cerebral hypoperfusion. This condition requires close monitoring and often valve replacement.

Q386. Answer: D

Explanation: Pink frothy sputum and acute dyspnea indicate pulmonary edema. Left ventricular failure leads to increased pulmonary capillary pressure. Fluid leaks into alveoli, impairing gas exchange. Rapid intervention with oxygen and diuretics is required. This represents acute decompensation of cardiac function.

Q387. Answer: B

Explanation: Vegetations from infected heart valves can embolize to cerebral arteries. This leads to sudden neurologic deficits consistent with stroke. Endocarditis increases risk of septic emboli. Immediate imaging and management are critical. The symptoms reflect vascular occlusion rather than metabolic disturbance.

Q388. Answer: D

Explanation: Chronic pressure overload stimulates myocardial hypertrophy. Thickening of the ventricular wall reduces wall stress according to Laplace's law. Initially, systolic function may remain preserved. Over time, stiffness leads to diastolic dysfunction. This adaptation eventually becomes maladaptive.

Q389. Answer: C

Explanation: Rest pain signifies severe reduction in arterial blood flow. Critical limb ischemia occurs when perfusion is insufficient even without exertion. This is a limb-threatening condition. Prompt vascular evaluation is required. The pain typically improves when the limb is dependent.

Q390. Answer: C

Explanation: Beta-blockers inhibit sympathetic stimulation of the heart. This decreases heart rate and contractility. While beneficial long term, excessive slowing may cause symptomatic bradycardia. Monitoring is necessary during dose titration. The primary action is reduction of adrenergic effects.

Q391. Answer: C

Explanation: Mitral stenosis obstructs blood flow from left atrium to ventricle. Elevated atrial pressure transmits backward to pulmonary veins. Chronic pulmonary venous hypertension leads to capillary rupture and hemoptysis. Dyspnea results from congestion. The issue originates from valvular obstruction.

Q392. Answer: C

Explanation: Severe myocardial dysfunction can reduce cardiac output. Hypotension leads to decreased cerebral blood flow. Confusion is a sign of systemic hypoperfusion. This presentation indicates cardiogenic shock. Immediate hemodynamic support is required.

Q393. Answer: A

Explanation: Atrial fibrillation eliminates coordinated atrial contraction. Loss of atrial kick decreases ventricular filling, especially in stiff ventricles. Cardiac output may decline. Symptoms include fatigue and dyspnea. Rate control improves hemodynamic stability.

Q394. Answer: A

Explanation: Positional chest pain suggests pericardial inflammation. A pericardial friction rub is a classic auscultatory finding. It results from inflamed pericardial layers rubbing together. The pain is typically sharp and pleuritic. Recognition guides anti-inflammatory treatment.

Q395. Answer: D

Explanation: Heart failure activates antidiuretic hormone and renin-angiotensin systems. Water retention dilutes serum sodium concentration. Hyponatremia indicates advanced disease severity. It reflects poor prognosis if persistent. Managing fluid balance can help correct levels.

Q396. Answer: B

Explanation: Pulseless ventricular tachycardia is a shockable rhythm. Immediate defibrillation restores organized electrical activity. Delayed treatment reduces survival chances. Advanced cardiac life support protocols prioritize early shock delivery.

Q397. Answer: A

Explanation: Retinal hemorrhages and papilledema indicate acute target organ damage. This presentation defines hypertensive emergency. Immediate controlled blood pressure reduction is required. Without treatment, risk of stroke or organ failure increases.

Q398. Answer: A

Explanation: Dilated cardiomyopathy involves enlargement of ventricular chambers. Contractile function is reduced, leading to systolic failure. Low cardiac output results in hypotension and fatigue. The structural defect is dilation rather than hypertrophy.

Q399. Answer: D

Explanation: Papillary muscle rupture is a mechanical complication of myocardial infarction. It leads to acute severe mitral regurgitation. Sudden pulmonary edema and new murmur are classic findings. Immediate surgical intervention is often required.

Q400. Answer: D

Explanation: Sodium intake influences water retention through renal mechanisms. Reducing sodium decreases intravascular volume. Lower preload reduces symptoms of congestion in heart failure. Dietary modification complements pharmacologic therapy. Consistent adherence improves symptom control.

Question (401-500)

Q401. A patient with acute inferior wall myocardial infarction develops hypotension and clear lung fields; which complication is most likely responsible?
(A) Right ventricular infarction
(B) Ventricular septal defect
(C) Left ventricular aneurysm
(D) Papillary muscle rupture

Q402. A patient on continuous heparin infusion shows a sudden drop in platelet count from 250,000/µL to 90,000/µL within five days; what is the priority action?
(A) Increase infusion rate
(B) Transfuse platelets
(C) Discontinue heparin immediately
(D) Administer protamine sulfate

Q403. A patient with chronic heart failure reports gaining 3 kg in two days; which assessment finding would most strongly correlate with fluid overload?
(A) Bradycardia
(B) Dry mucous membranes
(C) Elevated jugular venous pressure
(D) Hypoactive bowel sounds

Q404. During administration of alteplase for acute ischemic stroke, which parameter must be assessed before infusion?
(A) LDL cholesterol level
(B) Serum potassium level
(C) Hemoglobin A1c
(D) Time of symptom onset

Q405. A telemetry strip shows irregularly irregular rhythm without discernible P waves; what is the most likely rhythm?
(A) Atrial flutter
(B) Ventricular tachycardia
(C) Atrial fibrillation
(D) Sinus arrhythmia

Q406. A patient undergoing percutaneous coronary intervention develops sudden chest pain and hypotension; what is the immediate concern?
(A) Anxiety reaction
(B) Coronary artery dissection
(C) Electrolyte imbalance
(D) Hyperglycemia

Q407. A patient with peripheral arterial disease reports calf pain after walking 100 meters that resolves with rest; what mechanism explains this symptom?
(A) Neuropathic irritation
(B) Ischemia due to arterial narrowing
(C) Lymphatic obstruction
(D) Venous stasis

Q408. A patient receiving warfarin has an INR of 6.5 without bleeding; what is the appropriate management?
(A) Increase dose
(B) Administer vitamin K
(C) Start aspirin
(D) Continue same dose

Q409. A post-cardiac surgery patient develops muffled heart sounds and jugular venous distention; what complication is suspected?
(A) Pulmonary edema
(B) Cardiac tamponade
(C) Atelectasis
(D) Myocarditis

Q410. Which laboratory value is most specific for myocardial injury?
(A) CK-MB
(B) LDH
(C) Troponin I
(D) Myoglobin

Q411. A patient with hypertensive crisis presents with headache and blurred vision; what is the priority intervention?
(A) Gradual controlled blood pressure reduction
(B) Encourage ambulation
(C) Immediate diuretic bolus only
(D) Rapid reduction of blood pressure to normal

Q412. A patient with heart failure is prescribed spironolactone; which electrolyte imbalance is most concerning?
(A) Hypokalemia
(B) Hyponatremia
(C) Hyperkalemia
(D) Hypocalcemia

Q413. A patient with deep vein thrombosis suddenly develops dyspnea and chest pain; what is the likely diagnosis?
(A) Pulmonary embolism
(B) Pneumonia
(C) Myocardial infarction

(D) Pericarditis

Q414. Which lifestyle modification most effectively reduces cardiovascular risk?

(A) Limiting sleep
(B) Increased sodium intake
(C) High saturated fat diet
(D) Smoking cessation

Q415. A patient's ECG shows ST elevation in leads II, III, and aVF; which coronary artery is most likely occluded?

(A) Left anterior descending
(B) Diagonal branch
(C) Right coronary artery
(D) Left circumflex

Q416. A patient receiving digoxin reports visual halos and nausea; what is the most appropriate action?

(A) Check serum digoxin level
(B) Encourage fluid intake
(C) Administer next dose
(D) Give antacid

Q417. Which assessment finding indicates left-sided heart failure?

(A) Hepatomegaly
(B) Ascites
(C) Peripheral cyanosis only
(D) Pulmonary crackles

Q418. A patient with carotid artery stenosis is at highest risk for which complication?

(A) Deep vein thrombosis
(B) Stroke
(C) Pulmonary edema
(D) Renal failure

Q419. A patient undergoing cardioversion must have which intervention performed first?

(A) Chest physiotherapy
(B) Anticoagulation assessment
(C) Administration of antibiotics
(D) Fasting for 24 hours

Q420. Which finding most strongly suggests infective endocarditis?

(A) Bradycardia
(B) Hyperglycemia
(C) Elevated LDL
(D) Splinter hemorrhages

Q421. A patient with chronic hypertension presents with sudden tearing chest pain radiating to the back; which condition is most likely?

(A) Stable angina
(B) Pericarditis
(C) Pulmonary embolism
(D) Aortic dissection

Q422. A patient with heart failure is prescribed a low-sodium diet; what is the primary purpose of this intervention?

(A) Reduce fluid retention
(B) Increase cardiac contractility
(C) Improve oxygen saturation
(D) Prevent hypoglycemia

Q423. A patient develops chest discomfort relieved by sitting forward and worsened by inspiration; which diagnosis is most consistent?

(A) Heart block
(B) Pericarditis
(C) Myocardial infarction
(D) Stable angina

Q424. Which medication class is first-line therapy for reducing mortality in systolic heart failure?

(A) Antiplatelet agents
(B) Calcium channel blockers
(C) Nitrates only
(D) ACE inhibitors

Q425. A patient with atrial fibrillation complains of palpitations and dizziness; which complication is most concerning?

(A) Hyperlipidemia
(B) Anemia
(C) Stroke
(D) Hypoglycemia

Q426. A post-catheterization patient develops a rapidly expanding hematoma at the femoral site; what is the immediate action?

(A) Remove dressing
(B) Elevate the head of bed
(C) Encourage ambulation
(D) Apply firm manual pressure

Q427. A patient with mitral stenosis is most likely to experience which symptom?

(A) Sudden weight loss
(B) Hematuria
(C) Polyuria
(D) Dyspnea on exertion

Q428. A patient receiving beta-blockers should be monitored for which adverse effect?
(A) Tachycardia
(B) Hyperglycemia
(C) Bradycardia
(D) Hypertension
Q429. Which diagnostic test best evaluates left ventricular ejection fraction?
(A) Chest X-ray
(B) Electrolyte panel
(C) Stress ECG only
(D) Echocardiogram
Q430. A patient with acute coronary syndrome receives nitroglycerin; what is its primary mechanism of action?
(A) Decrease oxygen saturation
(B) Increase platelet aggregation
(C) Vasodilation of coronary arteries
(D) Increase heart rate
Q431. A patient with peripheral edema and ascites likely has dysfunction of which cardiac chamber?
(A) Left atrium
(B) Right ventricle
(C) Left ventricle
(D) Aortic valve
Q432. Which finding indicates successful thrombolytic therapy in myocardial infarction?
(A) ST-segment resolution
(B) Rising troponin levels only
(C) Decreased urine output
(D) Persistent chest pain
Q433. A patient with uncontrolled diabetes is at increased risk for which cardiovascular complication?
(A) Bradyarrhythmia
(B) Atherosclerosis
(C) Hypotension only
(D) Valve prolapse
Q434. Which intervention is most appropriate for a patient with symptomatic bradycardia and hypotension?
(A) Atropine administration
(B) Encourage rest only
(C) Immediate defibrillation
(D) Administer diuretics
Q435. A patient reports chest pain after emotional stress that resolves with rest; which condition is suggested?
(A) Pericardial effusion
(B) Stable angina
(C) Endocarditis
(D) Myocarditis
Q436. A patient with heart failure is advised to monitor daily weights; what is the rationale?
(A) Assess muscle mass
(B) Detect early fluid retention
(C) Measure bone density
(D) Evaluate metabolism
Q437. A patient presents with sudden unilateral weakness and slurred speech; which is the priority action?
(A) Administer insulin
(B) Initiate stroke protocol
(C) Encourage ambulation
(D) Provide oral fluids
Q438. A patient with infective endocarditis is at risk for which systemic complication?
(A) Hypothermia
(B) Polycythemia
(C) Hypercalcemia
(D) Septic emboli
Q439. Which electrolyte imbalance increases risk for ventricular arrhythmias?
(A) Hypercalcemia
(B) Hypernatremia
(C) Hypokalemia
(D) Hypermagnesemia
Q440. A patient undergoing valve replacement requires long-term anticoagulation; which complication is the primary concern?
(A) Dehydration
(B) Bleeding
(C) Infection only
(D) Hyperglycemia
Q441. A patient with dilated cardiomyopathy is most likely to exhibit which primary problem?
(A) Impaired ventricular contraction
(B) Decreased atrial size
(C) Increased ventricular wall thickness
(D) Valve calcification

Q442. A patient with acute pulmonary edema presents with severe dyspnea and frothy sputum; what is the priority intervention?
(A) Provide high-sodium meal
(B) Place patient in supine position
(C) Encourage oral fluids
(D) Administer oxygen therapy
Q443. A patient with unstable angina is admitted; what differentiates this condition from stable angina?
(A) Pain at rest or increasing frequency
(B) Relief with exercise
(C) Predictable pattern
(D) Pain only during exertion
Q444. A patient receiving amiodarone should have which function monitored regularly?
(A) Pancreatic enzymes
(B) Hemoglobin level
(C) Liver and thyroid function
(D) Renal function only
Q445. A patient with hypertension is advised to follow the DASH diet; what is its primary focus?
(A) High saturated fats
(B) Increased sodium intake
(C) High cholesterol foods
(D) Fruits, vegetables, and low-fat dairy
Q446. A patient presents with chest pain and diffuse ST elevation across multiple leads; what condition is most likely?
(A) Localized myocardial infarction
(B) Pericarditis
(C) Heart block
(D) Pulmonary embolism
Q447. A patient with heart failure reports orthopnea; what mechanism explains this symptom?
(A) Increased venous return when lying flat
(B) Reduced preload when supine
(C) Reduced systemic resistance
(D) Decreased pulmonary blood flow
Q448. A patient with atrial flutter typically shows which ECG finding?
(A) Absent QRS complexes
(B) Wide QRS only
(C) Irregular baseline without pattern
(D) Sawtooth flutter waves
Q449. A patient with severe aortic stenosis is most likely to experience which symptom triad?
(A) Edema, ascites, cyanosis
(B) Polyuria, thirst, fatigue
(C) Fever, rash, cough
(D) Chest pain, syncope, dyspnea
Q450. A patient with hyperlipidemia is prescribed a statin; what is the primary benefit?
(A) Raise blood glucose
(B) Increase clot formation
(C) Increase triglycerides
(D) Decrease LDL cholesterol
Q451. A patient presents with pulsus paradoxus; this finding is most associated with which condition?
(A) Hyperthyroidism
(B) Stable angina
(C) Hypertension
(D) Cardiac tamponade
Q452. A patient with ventricular tachycardia without a pulse requires which immediate intervention?
(A) Oxygen only
(B) Diuretics
(C) Defibrillation
(D) Atropine
Q453. A patient with chronic venous insufficiency should be instructed to do what to improve symptoms?
(A) Leg elevation
(B) Prolonged standing
(C) Restrict ambulation
(D) Apply heat continuously
Q454. A patient with metabolic syndrome has which combination of risk factors?
(A) Abdominal obesity, hypertension, insulin resistance
(B) Low blood pressure and anemia
(C) Hyperthyroidism and weight loss
(D) Bradycardia and hypotension
Q455. A patient taking furosemide should be monitored for which electrolyte imbalance?
(A) Hypernatremia
(B) Hypokalemia
(C) Hyperkalemia
(D) Hypercalcemia

Q456. A patient with myocardial infarction develops a new holosystolic murmur; what complication is suspected?
(A) Pericardial friction rub
(B) Ventricular septal rupture
(C) Hyperlipidemia
(D) Sinus bradycardia
Q457. A patient experiencing Raynaud phenomenon should avoid which trigger?
(A) Mild exercise
(B) Cold exposure
(C) Warm environments
(D) Adequate hydration
Q458. A patient with left bundle branch block may have difficulty diagnosing which condition on ECG?
(A) Inferior myocardial infarction
(B) Sinus tachycardia
(C) Atrial fibrillation
(D) ST-elevation myocardial infarction
Q459. A patient with cardiogenic shock will most likely exhibit which hemodynamic change?
(A) Increased cardiac output
(B) Increased urine output
(C) Decreased systemic vascular resistance
(D) Decreased cardiac output
Q460. A patient prescribed clopidogrel should be educated about which potential side effect?
(A) Increased bleeding
(B) Hypertension
(C) Hyperkalemia
(D) Bradycardia
Q461. A 62-year-old patient with a history of hypertension presents with sudden onset chest pressure radiating to the left arm while shoveling snow. The pain persists despite rest. What is the most appropriate immediate nursing action?
(A) Encourage deep breathing exercises
(B) Obtain a 12-lead ECG
(C) Schedule an outpatient stress test
(D) Advise the patient to take antacids
Q462. A patient with heart failure reports increasing shortness of breath at night and requires three pillows to sleep comfortably. Which intervention should the nurse prioritize?
(A) Increase sodium intake
(B) Limit fluid monitoring
(C) Encourage supine positioning
(D) Assess for pulmonary crackles
Q463. A postoperative coronary artery bypass patient suddenly develops confusion and right-sided weakness. What is the priority action?
(A) Document and reassess in one hour
(B) Activate stroke response protocol
(C) Administer analgesics
(D) Encourage oral intake
Q464. A patient receiving IV nitroglycerin develops a blood pressure of 82/50 mmHg. What should the nurse do first?
(A) Lower the head of the bed
(B) Administer diuretics
(C) Increase infusion rate
(D) Stop or reduce the infusion
Q465. A patient with atrial fibrillation and rapid ventricular response reports dizziness. Heart rate is 150 bpm. Which medication is most appropriate to control rate?
(A) Atropine
(B) Adenosine
(C) Epinephrine
(D) Diltiazem
Q466. A patient with peripheral arterial disease presents with a pale, cool foot and absent pedal pulse. What is the nurse's immediate concern?
(A) Cellulitis
(B) Chronic venous stasis
(C) Acute arterial occlusion
(D) Lymphedema
Q467. A patient on long-term warfarin therapy reports black tarry stools. What is the priority action?
(A) Reassure patient
(B) Continue medication
(C) Assess INR level
(D) Encourage high vitamin K diet
Q468. A patient with acute myocardial infarction develops frequent premature ventricular contractions. What is the priority intervention?
(A) Ignore if asymptomatic
(B) Assess serum potassium level
(C) Administer oral fluids

(D) Encourage ambulation

Q469. A patient with cardiomyopathy reports swelling of ankles and fatigue despite medication adherence. What should the nurse assess first?

(A) Hearing ability
(B) Dietary sodium intake
(C) Visual acuity
(D) Skin temperature

Q470. A patient collapses in the hospital corridor and is unresponsive with no pulse. What is the nurse's first action?

(A) Call family
(B) Begin chest compressions
(C) Check blood glucose
(D) Obtain blood pressure

Q471. A patient with severe mitral regurgitation reports increasing fatigue and dyspnea on exertion. What underlying mechanism explains these symptoms?

(A) Decreased pulmonary pressure
(B) Reduced right ventricular preload
(C) Increased systemic resistance only
(D) Backflow of blood into left atrium

Q472. A patient admitted for hypertensive emergency has blood pressure 220/120 mmHg with headache and visual disturbances. What is the priority goal?

(A) Normalize blood pressure immediately
(B) Reduce blood pressure gradually
(C) Encourage ambulation
(D) Provide high-sodium diet

Q473. A patient with heart failure has a BNP level significantly elevated. What does this indicate?

(A) Increased ventricular wall stress
(B) Improved ventricular function
(C) Dehydration
(D) Normal cardiac output

Q474. A patient receiving thrombolytic therapy suddenly develops severe headache and confusion. What is the priority action?

(A) Encourage rest
(B) Give analgesics
(C) Continue infusion
(D) Stop infusion and notify provider

Q475. A patient with chronic stable angina asks how to prevent episodes during exercise. What is the best advice?

(A) Avoid all physical activity
(B) Skip medications
(C) Increase sodium intake
(D) Take nitroglycerin before exertion

Q476. A patient with deep vein thrombosis is on bed rest. What complication is the nurse most concerned about?

(A) Bradycardia
(B) Hyperthyroidism
(C) Hypertension
(D) Pulmonary embolism

Q477. A patient recovering from myocardial infarction asks when to resume sexual activity. What is the best guidance?

(A) Never resume
(B) After six months
(C) Immediately upon discharge
(D) After climbing two flights of stairs without symptoms

Q478. A patient with heart block type II experiences syncope. What intervention is most appropriate?

(A) Permanent pacemaker evaluation
(B) Diuretic therapy
(C) Oral beta-blocker
(D) Increase fluid intake

Q479. A patient with abdominal aortic aneurysm reports sudden severe abdominal pain and hypotension. What is the priority action?

(A) Prepare for emergency surgery
(B) Schedule outpatient visit
(C) Encourage oral fluids
(D) Provide analgesics only

Q480. A patient with chronic heart failure is prescribed an exercise program. What is the expected benefit?

(A) Decrease cardiac efficiency
(B) Increase resting heart rate
(C) Improve functional capacity
(D) Promote fluid retention

Q481. A 58-year-old patient with a history of smoking presents with crushing chest pain and diaphoresis. The ECG shows ST elevation in

anterior leads. What is the priority nursing action?
(A) Obtain a lipid profile
(B) Administer sublingual nitroglycerin only
(C) Prepare for immediate reperfusion therapy
(D) Encourage the patient to rest quietly
Q482. A patient with chronic heart failure reports persistent cough with pink frothy sputum. What should the nurse suspect?
(A) Allergic reaction
(B) Dehydration
(C) Upper respiratory infection
(D) Acute pulmonary edema
Q483. A patient receiving beta-blocker therapy for hypertension reports dizziness when standing. What is the most appropriate assessment?
(A) Measure temperature
(B) Assess bowel sounds
(C) Evaluate hearing acuity
(D) Check for orthostatic hypotension
Q484. A patient with atrial fibrillation is scheduled for elective cardioversion. What must be confirmed before the procedure?
(A) Normal hemoglobin level
(B) Adequate anticoagulation status
(C) Recent chest X-ray
(D) Normal potassium intake
Q485. A patient with peripheral arterial disease reports pain at rest in the foot. What does this indicate?
(A) Improved circulation
(B) Muscle strain
(C) Venous insufficiency
(D) Progression to critical limb ischemia
Q486. A patient develops sudden shortness of breath after long-distance travel. Oxygen saturation is low and heart rate is elevated. What is the most likely diagnosis?
(A) Myocarditis
(B) Stable angina
(C) Asthma exacerbation
(D) Pulmonary embolism
Q487. A patient with severe aortic regurgitation complains of bounding pulses. What is the underlying cause?
(A) Increased diastolic pressure
(B) Reduced cardiac output only
(C) Wide pulse pressure
(D) Decreased stroke volume
Q488. A patient receiving IV heparin therapy has an aPTT below therapeutic range. What is the nurse's priority action?
(A) Increase infusion per protocol
(B) Stop infusion permanently
(C) Decrease infusion rate
(D) Administer vitamin K
Q489. A patient with left-sided heart failure experiences paroxysmal nocturnal dyspnea. What explains this symptom?
(A) Dehydration
(B) Decreased venous return during sleep
(C) Fluid redistribution to lungs at night
(D) Increased renal output
Q490. A patient undergoing carotid endarterectomy suddenly develops difficulty speaking postoperatively. What is the nurse's first action?
(A) Offer water
(B) Encourage ambulation
(C) Reassure patient
(D) Notify surgical team immediately
Q491. A patient with infective endocarditis reports flank pain and hematuria. What complication is suspected?
(A) Renal embolization
(B) Hypotension only
(C) Dehydration
(D) Hyperlipidemia
Q492. A patient with cardiogenic shock has cool clammy skin and decreased urine output. What is the primary goal of treatment?
(A) Increase cardiac output
(B) Promote sedation only
(C) Decrease oxygen therapy
(D) Increase fluid overload
Q493. A patient with hyperkalemia demonstrates peaked T waves on ECG. What is the immediate concern?
(A) Ventricular arrhythmias
(B) Hypoglycemia
(C) Hypertension
(D) Bradycardia only
Q494. A patient with coronary artery disease is prescribed aspirin daily. What is the primary purpose?

(A) Reduce blood pressure
(B) Prevent platelet aggregation
(C) Increase heart rate
(D) Lower cholesterol

Q495. A patient presents with sharp chest pain that worsens with inspiration and improves when leaning forward. What is the likely diagnosis?
(A) Pericarditis
(B) Pulmonary hypertension
(C) Cardiomyopathy
(D) Stable angina

Q496. A patient with uncontrolled hypertension develops blurred vision and epistaxis. What complication is most concerning?
(A) End-organ damage
(B) Hyperlipidemia
(C) Dehydration
(D) Asthma

Q497. A patient with heart failure is prescribed an ACE inhibitor. Which effect indicates therapeutic benefit?
(A) Increased heart rate
(B) Elevated potassium only
(C) Reduced ventricular remodeling
(D) Increased afterload

Q498. A patient with acute limb ischemia reports numbness and inability to move toes. What is the nurse's priority?
(A) Encourage ambulation
(B) Apply warm compress
(C) Elevate limb above heart
(D) Notify vascular surgeon immediately

Q499. A patient with chronic atrial fibrillation asks about stroke prevention. What is the most effective strategy?
(A) Increased caffeine intake
(B) Long-term anticoagulation therapy
(C) Daily multivitamin
(D) Bed rest

Q500. A patient with heart failure presents with sudden weight gain and ankle swelling despite medication compliance. What should the nurse reinforce?
(A) Avoid daily weights
(B) Increased sodium restriction
(C) Discontinuation of diuretics
(D) Increased fluid intake

Answer Key and Explanation (401-500)

Q401. Answer: A

Explanation: Inferior wall infarctions may extend to involve the right ventricle, leading to impaired right ventricular filling and reduced preload to the left ventricle. This results in hypotension with clear lung fields because pulmonary congestion is absent. The clinical hallmark includes elevated jugular venous pressure with systemic hypotension. Early recognition is critical because management differs from left-sided failure. Volume loading rather than aggressive diuresis is often required to maintain cardiac output.

Q402. Answer: C

Explanation: A rapid decline in platelet count after heparin exposure suggests heparin-induced thrombocytopenia, an immune-mediated reaction. Continuing therapy increases the risk of life-threatening thrombosis. Immediate discontinuation is required to prevent further complications. Alternative anticoagulation should be initiated if indicated. Early identification significantly reduces morbidity and mortality.

Q403. Answer: C

Explanation: Rapid weight gain in heart failure commonly reflects fluid retention rather than adipose accumulation. Elevated jugular venous pressure indicates increased central venous pressure and systemic congestion. This finding correlates with right-sided volume overload. Peripheral edema and pulmonary symptoms may also develop. Prompt intervention can prevent decompensation.

Q404. Answer: D

Explanation: Thrombolytic therapy effectiveness and safety depend on the time window since symptom onset. Administration beyond the recommended timeframe increases hemorrhagic risk. Accurate history ensures eligibility for treatment. Early intervention improves neurologic outcomes. Documentation of timing is a critical safety requirement.

Q405. Answer: C

Explanation: An irregularly irregular rhythm with absent distinct P waves is characteristic of atrial fibrillation. Chaotic atrial electrical activity prevents coordinated atrial contraction. This increases the risk of thromboembolism due to blood stasis. Rate control and anticoagulation are key management priorities. Early identification prevents stroke-related complications.

Q406. Answer: B

Explanation: Sudden hemodynamic instability during coronary intervention suggests mechanical complications. Coronary artery dissection can abruptly compromise blood flow. Rapid recognition is necessary to restore perfusion. Failure to intervene promptly may result in myocardial damage. Continuous monitoring during procedures is essential for early detection.

Q407. Answer: B

Explanation: Intermittent claudication results from reduced arterial blood flow during exertion. Muscle oxygen demand increases with activity but cannot be met due to narrowed arteries. Rest decreases demand, relieving pain. This pattern is classic for peripheral arterial disease. Progressive symptoms may indicate worsening obstruction.

Q408. Answer: B

Explanation: A significantly elevated INR increases bleeding risk even in absence of symptoms. Vitamin K helps reverse excessive anticoagulation. Temporary cessation of therapy is typically indicated. Close monitoring ensures safe therapeutic adjustment. Prompt action prevents hemorrhagic complications.

Q409. Answer: B

Explanation: Muffled heart sounds combined with jugular venous distention suggest fluid accumulation in the pericardial space. Cardiac tamponade restricts ventricular filling and reduces cardiac output. Hypotension may also be present as part of the classic triad. Rapid intervention is life-saving. Emergent pericardiocentesis is often required.

Q410. Answer: C

Explanation: Troponin I is highly specific for myocardial cell injury and remains elevated for several days. It provides superior diagnostic accuracy compared to older markers. Serial measurements help confirm evolving infarction.

Elevated levels correlate with prognosis. Timely interpretation guides therapeutic decisions.

Q411. Answer: A

Explanation: In hypertensive crisis, overly rapid blood pressure reduction can cause cerebral hypoperfusion. Controlled, gradual lowering prevents end-organ damage while maintaining adequate perfusion. Continuous monitoring is required. Intravenous antihypertensives are commonly used. Careful titration minimizes complications.

Q412. Answer: C

Explanation: Spironolactone is a potassium-sparing diuretic that reduces aldosterone effects. Potassium retention can lead to dangerous elevations. Hyperkalemia may precipitate arrhythmias. Monitoring serum potassium is essential during therapy. Patient education regarding diet and supplements is important.

Q413. Answer: A

Explanation: A thrombus from the deep veins can dislodge and travel to pulmonary arteries. This blocks blood flow and impairs oxygenation. Sudden dyspnea and pleuritic chest pain are classic symptoms. Prompt diagnostic imaging and anticoagulation are critical. Untreated cases can rapidly become fatal.

Q414. Answer: D

Explanation: Smoking damages vascular endothelium and accelerates atherosclerosis. Cessation significantly lowers cardiovascular morbidity and mortality. Benefits begin shortly after quitting and continue long term. Risk reduction exceeds many pharmacologic interventions. Comprehensive support improves cessation success.

Q415. Answer: C

Explanation: Leads II, III, and aVF reflect the inferior wall of the heart. Inferior infarctions commonly result from right coronary artery occlusion. Correlating ECG findings with anatomy guides intervention. Early reperfusion limits myocardial damage. Prompt recognition improves survival outcomes.

Q416. Answer: A

Explanation: Visual disturbances and gastrointestinal symptoms are classic signs of digoxin toxicity. Serum level assessment confirms suspected toxicity. Renal function and electrolyte status should also be evaluated. Early detection prevents serious arrhythmias. Dose adjustment may be required.

Q417. Answer: D

Explanation: Left-sided heart failure leads to pulmonary congestion due to impaired left ventricular output. Fluid backs up into pulmonary circulation. Crackles on auscultation reflect alveolar fluid accumulation. Patients may also experience dyspnea and orthopnea. Early management reduces respiratory compromise.

Q418. Answer: B

Explanation: Carotid artery narrowing can reduce cerebral perfusion or release emboli. This significantly increases stroke risk. Transient ischemic attacks may precede major events. Early detection and management lower morbidity. Surgical or medical therapy may be indicated.

Q419. Answer: B

Explanation: Cardioversion can dislodge atrial thrombi, leading to embolic stroke. Assessing anticoagulation status minimizes this risk. Adequate anticoagulation is typically required before elective procedures. Transesophageal echocardiography may be used to rule out thrombus. Safety protocols reduce complications.

Q420. Answer: D

Explanation: Splinter hemorrhages are small linear bleeding lesions under the nails associated with microemboli. Infective endocarditis can produce septic emboli and vascular phenomena. Fever and heart murmur are also common findings. Blood cultures aid diagnosis. Early antimicrobial therapy is essential.

Q421. Answer: D

Explanation: Sudden severe chest pain described as tearing and radiating to the back is classic for aortic dissection. This condition involves separation of the layers of the aortic wall. It is life-threatening and requires immediate intervention. Blood pressure control is critical to prevent extension. Early imaging confirms the diagnosis and guides surgical management.

Q422. Answer: A

Explanation: Sodium promotes water retention, which can worsen fluid overload in heart failure. Restricting sodium helps reduce edema and pulmonary congestion. This decreases cardiac workload and improves symptoms. Dietary management is a cornerstone of chronic heart failure care. Patient education ensures long-term adherence.

Q423. Answer: B

Explanation: Positional chest pain that improves when leaning forward suggests pericardial inflammation. Inflammation of the pericardial sac causes friction and irritation. Pain often worsens with deep breathing or lying supine. A pericardial friction rub may be auscultated. Early treatment reduces risk of complications such as effusion.

Q424. Answer: D

Explanation: ACE inhibitors reduce afterload and inhibit maladaptive remodeling in systolic dysfunction. They improve survival and decrease hospitalization rates. These agents are foundational in guideline-directed therapy. Monitoring renal function and potassium is necessary. Long-term adherence provides significant prognostic benefit.

Q425. Answer: C

Explanation: Atrial fibrillation predisposes to clot formation in the atria due to ineffective contraction. Embolization of thrombi can lead to ischemic stroke. Dizziness may indicate reduced cerebral perfusion. Anticoagulation therapy reduces thromboembolic risk. Risk stratification tools guide management decisions.

Q426. Answer: D

Explanation: Expanding hematoma indicates active bleeding at the access site. Immediate manual compression prevents further blood loss. Monitoring vital signs is also essential. Delay can lead to hypovolemia or shock. Early intervention minimizes complications.

Q427. Answer: D

Explanation: Mitral stenosis obstructs blood flow from left atrium to left ventricle. This causes pulmonary congestion and exertional dyspnea. Over time, atrial enlargement may occur. Patients may also develop fatigue due to reduced cardiac output. Early management alleviates symptom progression.

Q428. Answer: C

Explanation: Beta-blockers reduce heart rate and myocardial contractility. Excessive slowing can result in symptomatic bradycardia. Monitoring pulse before administration is essential. Dose adjustments may be necessary in vulnerable patients. Patient education enhances safe medication use.

Q429. Answer: D

Explanation: Echocardiography provides real-time imaging of cardiac structure and function. It accurately measures ejection fraction and wall motion abnormalities. This helps assess severity of heart failure. It is noninvasive and widely available. Serial assessments monitor disease progression.

Q430. Answer: C

Explanation: Nitroglycerin causes smooth muscle relaxation leading to vasodilation. Coronary artery dilation improves myocardial oxygen supply. It also reduces preload, decreasing oxygen demand. This relieves ischemic chest pain. Monitoring blood pressure is important due to hypotension risk.

Q431. Answer: B

Explanation: Right ventricular failure leads to systemic venous congestion. This manifests as peripheral edema and ascites. Elevated venous pressures impair fluid return. Jugular venous distention may also be present. Management focuses on reducing volume overload.

Q432. Answer: A

Explanation: Resolution of ST-segment elevation suggests restored coronary perfusion. Clinical improvement often accompanies ECG changes. Early reperfusion limits infarct size. Serial ECG monitoring is essential. Biomarker trends also assist in evaluating response.

Q433. Answer: B

Explanation: Chronic hyperglycemia damages vascular endothelium. This accelerates plaque formation and atherosclerosis. Increased risk of coronary artery disease follows. Strict glycemic control reduces macrovascular complications. Comprehensive risk management is necessary.

Q434. Answer: A

Explanation: Symptomatic bradycardia can reduce cardiac output significantly. Atropine increases heart rate by blocking vagal stimulation. Prompt administration stabilizes hemodynamics. Continuous monitoring is required. Further interventions may be necessary if unresponsive.

Q435. Answer: B

Explanation: Stable angina occurs when myocardial oxygen demand exceeds supply during exertion or stress. Symptoms resolve with rest as demand decreases. This pattern indicates fixed coronary obstruction. Early treatment prevents progression. Risk factor modification is essential.

Q436. Answer: B

Explanation: Sudden weight gain often indicates fluid accumulation. Early detection allows timely intervention. This prevents hospitalization for decompensation. Consistent timing enhances accuracy. Patient self-monitoring improves outcomes.

Q437. Answer: B

Explanation: Acute neurologic deficits suggest possible stroke. Rapid activation of stroke protocol ensures timely imaging and treatment. Early intervention reduces permanent disability. Time-sensitive therapies depend on prompt recognition. Coordinated team response improves survival.

Q438. Answer: D

Explanation: Vegetations on heart valves can dislodge and travel systemically. These emboli may cause infarction in various organs. Persistent infection also damages cardiac structures. Blood cultures guide antimicrobial therapy. Early management prevents severe outcomes.

Q439. Answer: C

Explanation: Potassium is critical for cardiac electrical stability. Low levels prolong repolarization and increase excitability. This predisposes to ventricular arrhythmias. Monitoring is especially important in patients on diuretics. Prompt correction reduces risk.

Q440. Answer: B

Explanation: Anticoagulation reduces thromboembolic risk but increases bleeding tendency. Monitoring coagulation parameters ensures therapeutic balance. Patient education about signs of bleeding is essential. Regular follow-up improves safety. Early detection prevents severe hemorrhage.

Q441. Answer: A

Explanation: Dilated cardiomyopathy is characterized by enlargement of the ventricular chambers and reduced systolic function. The weakened myocardium cannot contract effectively, leading to decreased cardiac output. Patients often present with symptoms of heart failure such as fatigue and dyspnea. Ventricular dilation further worsens mechanical efficiency. Early treatment focuses on improving contractility and preventing remodeling.

Q442. Answer: D

Explanation: Acute pulmonary edema impairs oxygen exchange due to fluid accumulation in alveoli. Immediate oxygen administration improves tissue oxygenation. Positioning upright can also reduce pulmonary congestion. Rapid management prevents respiratory failure. Diuretics and vasodilators are often administered subsequently.

Q443. Answer: A

Explanation: Unstable angina presents with chest pain that may occur at rest or with minimal exertion. The pattern is often new or worsening compared to previous episodes. This indicates increased risk of myocardial infarction. Immediate evaluation and management are necessary. It represents an acute coronary syndrome.

Q444. Answer: C

Explanation: Amiodarone affects multiple organ systems including liver and thyroid. Regular monitoring detects toxicity early. Thyroid dysfunction may occur due to iodine content. Hepatic enzyme elevation is also possible. Long-term therapy requires comprehensive surveillance.

Q445. Answer: D

Explanation: The DASH diet emphasizes nutrient-rich foods such as fruits and vegetables. It limits sodium and saturated fats to control blood pressure. Increased potassium and fiber intake contribute to cardiovascular health. Clinical studies demonstrate significant reductions in blood pressure. Lifestyle changes complement pharmacologic therapy.

Q446. Answer: B

Explanation: Diffuse ST-segment elevation in multiple leads is characteristic of pericarditis. Unlike localized infarction, changes are widespread. Patients may also have PR segment depression. Clinical correlation includes pleuritic chest pain. Anti-inflammatory therapy is commonly indicated.

Q447. Answer: A

Explanation: When lying flat, venous return increases and exacerbates pulmonary congestion in heart failure. Fluid shifts from peripheral tissues into central circulation. This worsens shortness of breath. Elevating the head reduces symptoms. Orthopnea indicates worsening cardiac function.

Q448. Answer: D

Explanation: Atrial flutter produces rapid atrial depolarizations that appear as sawtooth waves on ECG. Ventricular response may be regular or variable. It differs from atrial fibrillation due to organized atrial activity. Rate control and rhythm management are essential. Anticoagulation may also be necessary.

Q449. Answer: D

Explanation: Severe aortic stenosis reduces blood flow from the left ventricle. Classic symptoms include angina, syncope, and dyspnea on exertion. Reduced cerebral perfusion contributes to fainting episodes. Left ventricular hypertrophy may develop. Valve replacement is often required in advanced disease.

Q450. Answer: D

Explanation: Statins inhibit cholesterol synthesis in the liver. This reduces LDL levels and slows plaque progression. They also stabilize atherosclerotic plaques. Reduced LDL significantly lowers cardiovascular event risk. Monitoring liver enzymes is recommended.

Q451. Answer: D

Explanation: Pulsus paradoxus refers to an exaggerated drop in systolic blood pressure during inspiration. It is commonly seen in cardiac tamponade. Pericardial fluid restricts ventricular filling. This leads to hemodynamic compromise. Immediate evaluation is essential.

Q452. Answer: C

Explanation: Pulseless ventricular tachycardia is a life-threatening arrhythmia. Immediate defibrillation restores organized cardiac rhythm. Delay reduces survival probability. Cardiopulmonary resuscitation should continue until shock delivery. Rapid response is critical.

Q453. Answer: A

Explanation: Elevating the legs promotes venous return and reduces edema. Chronic venous insufficiency results from impaired valve function. Swelling and skin changes may occur. Compression therapy may also help. Lifestyle modifications improve comfort and prevent ulcers.

Q454. Answer: A

Explanation: Metabolic syndrome involves a cluster of cardiovascular risk factors. Central obesity, hypertension, and insulin resistance are key components. Dyslipidemia is often present. This combination significantly increases cardiovascular risk. Lifestyle modification is essential for prevention.

Q455. Answer: B

Explanation: Furosemide is a loop diuretic that increases potassium excretion. Low potassium levels may lead to arrhythmias. Regular monitoring prevents complications. Dietary counseling may be required. Supplementation is sometimes necessary.

Q456. Answer: B

Explanation: A new murmur after myocardial infarction may indicate mechanical complications. Ventricular septal rupture causes abnormal blood flow between ventricles. This leads to acute heart failure and hemodynamic instability. Immediate evaluation is required. Surgical repair is often necessary.

Q457. Answer: B

Explanation: Raynaud phenomenon involves vasospasm of peripheral arteries. Cold exposure precipitates episodes. Fingers may turn white or blue due to reduced blood flow. Avoiding triggers reduces symptom frequency. Protective clothing is recommended.

Q458. Answer: D

Explanation: Left bundle branch block alters normal ventricular depolarization patterns. This can obscure ST-segment changes. Diagnosing acute myocardial infarction becomes challenging. Additional criteria may be required. Clinical correlation is essential.

Q459. Answer: D

Explanation: Cardiogenic shock results from severe pump failure. Cardiac output falls, leading to inadequate tissue perfusion. Hypotension and oliguria may develop. Compensatory vasoconstriction increases systemic resistance. Early intervention improves survival.

Q460. Answer: A

Explanation: Clopidogrel inhibits platelet aggregation to prevent thrombosis. This increases bleeding risk. Patients should report unusual bruising or bleeding. Regular monitoring enhances safety. Education supports medication adherence.

Q461. Answer: B

Explanation: Persistent chest pressure unrelieved by rest suggests an acute coronary syndrome. Immediate ECG acquisition is essential to identify ST changes or arrhythmias. Early detection enables rapid reperfusion therapy if indicated. Time-sensitive management significantly reduces myocardial damage. Prompt assessment improves survival outcomes.

Q462. Answer: D

Explanation: Worsening orthopnea suggests fluid accumulation in the lungs. Auscultation for crackles helps evaluate pulmonary congestion severity. Early identification allows timely medication adjustment. Diuretic therapy may need modification. Monitoring prevents acute decompensation.

Q463. Answer: B

Explanation: Acute neurologic deficits after cardiac surgery may indicate stroke. Rapid activation of stroke protocol ensures immediate imaging and evaluation. Early intervention reduces long-term disability. Delays can result in irreversible damage. Coordinated team response is critical.

Q464. Answer: D

Explanation: Nitroglycerin causes vasodilation and can lead to hypotension. Severe blood pressure reduction compromises organ perfusion. The infusion should be reduced or discontinued immediately. Monitoring vital signs is essential. Stabilization prevents shock progression.

Q465. Answer: D

Explanation: Rapid ventricular response reduces cardiac output and causes symptoms. Calcium channel blockers help slow atrioventricular conduction. Rate control improves hemodynamic stability. Continuous monitoring is necessary during administration. Effective control decreases complications.

Q466. Answer: C

Explanation: Sudden pallor, coolness, and absent pulse indicate impaired arterial perfusion. Acute occlusion threatens limb viability. Rapid intervention is required to restore circulation. Delayed treatment may result in tissue necrosis. Emergency evaluation is critical.

Q467. Answer: C

Explanation: Black tarry stools suggest gastrointestinal bleeding. Warfarin increases bleeding risk, especially if INR is elevated. Immediate laboratory assessment determines anticoagulation status. Dose adjustment or reversal may be necessary. Early action prevents severe hemorrhage.

Q468. Answer: B

Explanation: Ventricular ectopy after myocardial infarction may indicate electrical instability. Electrolyte imbalance, especially low potassium, increases arrhythmia risk. Identifying and correcting abnormalities reduces progression to ventricular tachycardia. Continuous monitoring is required. Early correction improves safety.

Q469. Answer: B

Explanation: Persistent edema often results from excessive sodium consumption. Even with medication compliance, dietary indiscretion can worsen fluid retention. Assessment identifies modifiable factors. Reinforcement of dietary education may be required. Early intervention prevents hospitalization.

Q470. Answer: B

Explanation: Absence of pulse indicates cardiac arrest. Immediate high-quality chest compressions maintain circulation. Early CPR improves survival outcomes. Defibrillation should follow if indicated. Rapid initiation is essential.

Q471. Answer: D

Explanation: Mitral regurgitation allows blood to flow backward during systole. This reduces forward cardiac output. Increased left atrial pressure leads to pulmonary congestion. Over time, ventricular dilation may occur. Symptoms reflect decreased efficiency of circulation.

Q472. Answer: B

Explanation: Rapid normalization can compromise cerebral perfusion. Controlled reduction prevents further end-organ damage. Intravenous medications are titrated carefully. Continuous monitoring is required. Gradual decrease improves safety.

Q473. Answer: A

Explanation: BNP is released in response to ventricular stretching. Elevated levels correlate with heart failure severity. It assists in diagnosis and monitoring. Higher values often reflect fluid overload. Treatment effectiveness may reduce levels.

Q474. Answer: D

Explanation: Sudden neurologic changes during thrombolytic therapy suggest intracranial bleeding. Immediate discontinuation reduces further risk. Rapid evaluation is essential. Early detection improves outcomes. Safety protocols must be followed strictly.

Q475. Answer: D

Explanation: Prophylactic nitroglycerin reduces myocardial oxygen demand during activity. It dilates coronary vessels and decreases preload. This prevents predictable angina episodes. Exercise remains important but should be moderated. Medication adherence improves quality of life.

Q476. Answer: D

Explanation: Immobility increases risk of thrombus dislodgement. A clot traveling to the lungs can obstruct pulmonary circulation. This is a life-threatening emergency. Monitoring respiratory status is essential. Anticoagulation reduces risk.

Q477. Answer: D

Explanation: Ability to tolerate moderate physical activity indicates readiness. Sexual activity requires similar exertion levels. Gradual resumption ensures safety. Open communication reduces anxiety. Education supports recovery.

Q478. Answer: A

Explanation: Type II heart block can progress unpredictably. Syncope indicates inadequate cerebral perfusion. Pacemaker therapy stabilizes heart rate. Early evaluation prevents sudden deterioration. Long-term pacing may be required.

Q479. Answer: A

Explanation: Sudden pain with hypotension suggests aneurysm rupture. This is a life-threatening emergency. Immediate surgical intervention is required. Delays increase mortality. Rapid stabilization and transfer are critical.

Q480. Answer: C

Explanation: Structured exercise improves cardiovascular endurance. It enhances peripheral oxygen utilization. Functional capacity increases over time. Symptoms such as fatigue may decrease. Supervised programs ensure safety and effectiveness.

Q481. Answer: C

Explanation: ST elevation in anterior leads indicates acute transmural myocardial injury. Rapid reperfusion therapy such as percutaneous coronary intervention is essential to restore blood flow. Delays increase myocardial necrosis and mortality. Early coordination with the cardiac team improves outcomes. Time-sensitive intervention is critical in ST-elevation myocardial infarction.

Q482. Answer: D

Explanation: Pink frothy sputum is a hallmark of pulmonary edema due to fluid leakage into alveoli. This condition results from increased pulmonary capillary pressure. It impairs oxygen exchange and may progress rapidly. Immediate assessment and oxygen support are necessary. Prompt diuretic therapy often follows stabilization.

Q483. Answer: D

Explanation: Beta-blockers can contribute to orthostatic hypotension. Dizziness upon standing suggests a drop in blood pressure with position change. Measuring blood pressure in supine and standing positions confirms the diagnosis. Adjusting medication or educating about slow position changes may be necessary. Preventing falls is a priority.

Q484. Answer: B

Explanation: Cardioversion may dislodge atrial thrombi formed during atrial fibrillation. Ensuring adequate anticoagulation reduces stroke risk. Therapeutic anticoagulation is typically required for several weeks prior. Alternatively, imaging may confirm absence of thrombus. Safety evaluation is essential before proceeding.

Q485. Answer: D

Explanation: Rest pain indicates severe arterial insufficiency. It suggests minimal blood flow even without exertion. This is a sign of advanced disease. Tissue viability may be compromised. Immediate vascular evaluation is necessary to prevent limb loss.

Q486. Answer: D

Explanation: Prolonged immobility during travel increases risk of deep vein thrombosis. A dislodged clot may travel to the pulmonary arteries. Sudden dyspnea and hypoxia are typical findings. Early anticoagulation improves survival. Prompt imaging confirms diagnosis.

Q487. Answer: C

Explanation: Aortic regurgitation allows blood to flow back into the left ventricle during diastole. This lowers diastolic pressure and increases systolic output. The resulting wide pulse pressure creates bounding pulses. Chronic volume overload may enlarge the ventricle. Surgical intervention may be required in severe cases.

Q488. Answer: A

Explanation: Subtherapeutic aPTT indicates inadequate anticoagulation. Increasing infusion according to protocol helps reach therapeutic levels. Proper anticoagulation prevents thrombus extension. Frequent monitoring ensures safe dosing adjustments. Protocol-driven care enhances patient safety.

Q489. Answer: C

Explanation: Lying flat increases venous return and redistributes peripheral fluid centrally. In heart failure, this worsens pulmonary congestion. Patients awaken suddenly with breathlessness. Sitting upright relieves symptoms. It indicates worsening ventricular dysfunction.

Q490. Answer: D

Explanation: New speech difficulty may indicate cerebral ischemia or stroke. Immediate notification allows rapid assessment and intervention. Early treatment reduces permanent deficits. Postoperative neurologic monitoring is essential. Prompt response improves outcomes.

Q491. Answer: A

Explanation: Vegetations from infected valves can embolize systemically. Renal emboli may cause flank pain and blood in urine. Early recognition prevents further organ damage. Blood cultures guide therapy. Prolonged antibiotic treatment is often required.

Q492. Answer: A

Explanation: Cardiogenic shock results from inadequate cardiac pump function. Increasing cardiac output improves tissue perfusion. Inotropic agents may be required. Monitoring urine output assesses renal perfusion. Early aggressive management reduces mortality.

Q493. Answer: A

Explanation: Elevated potassium affects cardiac conduction. Peaked T waves are early ECG changes. Severe hyperkalemia can progress to life-threatening arrhythmias. Rapid treatment stabilizes myocardial membranes. Continuous monitoring is essential.

Q494. Answer: B

Explanation: Aspirin inhibits platelet activation and aggregation. This reduces risk of clot formation in coronary arteries. It decreases incidence of myocardial infarction. Low-dose therapy provides antithrombotic benefit. Long-term adherence improves cardiovascular outcomes.

Q495. Answer: A

Explanation: Positional and pleuritic chest pain suggests inflammation of the pericardium. Leaning forward reduces pressure on the inflamed sac. Diffuse ECG changes may accompany symptoms. Early anti-inflammatory therapy prevents complications. Monitoring for effusion is important.

Q496. Answer: A

Explanation: Severe hypertension can damage organs such as brain, eyes, and kidneys. Blurred vision and nosebleeds suggest vascular stress. Immediate evaluation prevents progression. Gradual blood pressure reduction is required. Ongoing control reduces long-term risks.

Q497. Answer: C

Explanation: ACE inhibitors block angiotensin II production. This decreases vasoconstriction and prevents maladaptive remodeling. Over time, ventricular function stabilizes. Mortality and hospitalization rates decline. Monitoring ensures safe dosing.

Q498. Answer: D

Explanation: Neurologic deficits indicate severe ischemia. Tissue viability is threatened. Immediate surgical evaluation is necessary. Delayed treatment may result in amputation. Rapid restoration of blood flow is critical.

Q499. Answer: B

Explanation: Atrial fibrillation promotes clot formation in the atria. Anticoagulation significantly lowers stroke risk. Risk assessment tools guide therapy selection. Regular monitoring ensures therapeutic levels. Preventive strategy reduces morbidity.

Q500. Answer: B

Explanation: Fluid retention is commonly triggered by excessive sodium intake. Reinforcing strict dietary adherence helps control symptoms. Even small increases can worsen edema. Ongoing education promotes self-management. Early correction prevents hospitalization.

Question (501-600)

Q501. Which pathophysiologic mechanism primarily contributes to the development of left ventricular hypertrophy in chronic hypertension?

(A) Persistent pressure overload
(B) Increased venous capacitance
(C) Reduced preload
(D) Decreased systemic vascular resistance

Q502. What is the primary reason atrial fibrillation increases the risk of thromboembolic stroke?

(A) Increased coronary perfusion
(B) Enhanced ventricular contractility
(C) Reduced systemic blood flow
(D) Stasis of blood in the atria

Q503. Why does myocardial ischemia commonly produce chest pain during exertion?

(A) Enhanced parasympathetic activity
(B) Increased coronary vasodilation
(C) Imbalance between oxygen supply and demand
(D) Decreased oxygen demand

Q504. Which structural change most directly contributes to systolic heart failure?

(A) Increased atrial size only
(B) Impaired myocardial contractility
(C) Reduced systemic venous return
(D) Decreased ventricular compliance

Q505. What is the primary physiologic effect of ACE inhibitors in cardiovascular disease?

(A) Reduced vasoconstriction
(B) Increased angiotensin II production
(C) Enhanced sodium retention
(D) Elevated heart rate

Q506. How does hyperlipidemia accelerate atherosclerosis?

(A) Increases HDL levels
(B) Reduces inflammatory response
(C) Promotes endothelial repair
(D) Encourages lipid deposition in arterial walls

Q507. What explains the development of pulmonary edema in left-sided heart failure?

(A) Reduced pulmonary capillary pressure
(B) Elevated left atrial pressure
(C) Decreased venous return
(D) Increased lymphatic drainage

Q508. Why are beta-blockers beneficial after myocardial infarction?

(A) Promote vasoconstriction
(B) Decrease heart rate and workload
(C) Enhance platelet aggregation
(D) Increase myocardial oxygen consumption

Q509. What is the conceptual basis for using anticoagulation in deep vein thrombosis?

(A) Prevent clot extension and embolization
(B) Dissolve existing clots immediately
(C) Stimulate vasodilation only
(D) Increase platelet production

Q510. Why does severe aortic stenosis lead to syncope during exertion?

(A) Elevated venous return
(B) Reduced cerebral perfusion
(C) Increased diastolic filling time
(D) Excessive pulmonary blood flow

Q511. What mechanism explains the development of edema in right-sided heart failure?

(A) Reduced capillary permeability
(B) Elevated systemic venous pressure
(C) Increased renal perfusion
(D) Decreased systemic venous pressure

Q512. Why is time to treatment critical in ST-elevation myocardial infarction?

(A) Prolonged ischemia leads to irreversible necrosis
(B) Cardiac output increases automatically
(C) Coronary arteries dilate spontaneously
(D) Myocardial cells regenerate rapidly

Q513. What is the fundamental cause of ventricular arrhythmias in electrolyte imbalance?

(A) Increased oxygen delivery
(B) Altered myocardial conduction properties
(C) Enhanced valve function
(D) Reduced systemic resistance

Q514. Why does chronic smoking increase cardiovascular risk?

(A) Decreases platelet activity
(B) Causes vasodilation
(C) Damages vascular endothelium
(D) Improves endothelial integrity

Q515. What principle underlies the use of diuretics in heart failure management?

(A) Reduce fluid volume and congestion

(B) Promote sodium retention
(C) Enhance myocardial contractility
(D) Increase preload

Q516. Why is left bundle branch block significant in cardiac assessment?
(A) It increases cardiac output
(B) It may mask ischemic changes
(C) It enhances ventricular synchrony
(D) It reduces heart rate

Q517. What is the rationale for statin therapy in primary prevention?
(A) Elevate LDL cholesterol
(B) Stabilize atherosclerotic plaques
(C) Reduce heart rate
(D) Increase blood viscosity

Q518. Why does pericardial tamponade impair cardiac output?
(A) Compresses cardiac chambers
(B) Reduces venous pressure
(C) Increases ventricular filling
(D) Enhances myocardial contractility

Q519. What is the primary conceptual goal of cardiac rehabilitation?
(A) Restore functional capacity safely
(B) Promote bed rest
(C) Eliminate medication use
(D) Limit all physical activity

Q520. Why does insulin resistance contribute to cardiovascular disease?
(A) Reduces inflammatory markers
(B) Lowers blood pressure
(C) Promotes endothelial dysfunction
(D) Decreases triglyceride levels

Q521. A 64-year-old patient with a history of coronary artery disease arrives at the emergency department complaining of crushing substernal chest pain lasting 40 minutes. The pain radiates to the jaw and is associated with nausea. Vital signs show BP 150/90 mmHg and HR 104 bpm. What is the nurse's priority action?
(A) Obtain a 12-lead ECG immediately
(B) Administer oral antacid
(C) Schedule stress testing
(D) Encourage deep breathing

Q522. A 70-year-old patient with chronic heart failure reports a 2.5 kg weight gain over three days and increasing ankle swelling. Lung auscultation reveals bibasilar crackles. What is the most appropriate nursing intervention?
(A) Encourage fluid intake
(B) Discontinue diuretics
(C) Advise strict bed rest
(D) Reinforce low-sodium diet adherence

Q523. A 55-year-old patient recovering from myocardial infarction suddenly develops shortness of breath and pink frothy sputum. Oxygen saturation is 84%. What is the priority action?
(A) Offer oral fluids
(B) Place patient flat
(C) Administer high-flow oxygen
(D) Provide analgesics

Q524. A patient with atrial fibrillation is not taking prescribed anticoagulation and presents with sudden right-sided weakness and slurred speech. What is the most likely diagnosis?
(A) Seizure
(B) Migraine aura
(C) Ischemic stroke
(D) Hypoglycemia

Q525. A patient undergoing femoral artery catheterization reports severe back pain and dizziness post-procedure. Blood pressure is 88/60 mmHg. What complication is suspected?
(A) Dehydration
(B) Anxiety reaction
(C) Retroperitoneal bleeding
(D) Urinary retention

Q526. A 60-year-old patient with hypertension presents with severe headache, blurred vision, and BP 230/120 mmHg. What is the primary treatment goal?
(A) Provide high-sodium diet
(B) Rapid normalization of BP
(C) Gradual controlled reduction of BP
(D) Encourage ambulation

Q527. A patient with deep vein thrombosis suddenly develops sharp chest pain and tachypnea. What should the nurse suspect?
(A) Stable angina
(B) Asthma
(C) Pulmonary embolism
(D) Pneumonia

Q528. A patient with severe aortic stenosis reports syncope during physical activity. What explains this symptom?
(A) Inadequate cerebral blood flow
(B) Increased coronary perfusion
(C) Hyperglycemia
(D) Elevated pulmonary pressure
Q529. A 68-year-old patient presents with tearing chest pain radiating to the back and unequal blood pressures in both arms. What is the most likely diagnosis?
(A) Stable angina
(B) Pericarditis
(C) Gastroesophageal reflux
(D) Aortic dissection
Q530. A patient with heart failure is taking spironolactone and reports muscle weakness. Laboratory results show potassium 6.2 mEq/L. What is the nurse's priority?
(A) Notify provider immediately
(B) Restrict fluids only
(C) Continue medication
(D) Encourage potassium-rich foods
Q531. A patient with mitral regurgitation develops worsening fatigue and dyspnea. Echocardiogram shows left atrial enlargement. What mechanism explains this change?
(A) Backflow into left atrium
(B) Decreased venous return
(C) Reduced ventricular filling
(D) Forward flow obstruction
Q532. A patient collapses and monitor shows ventricular fibrillation. What is the first intervention?
(A) Administer atropine
(B) Defibrillate immediately
(C) Provide oxygen only
(D) Start IV fluids
Q533. A patient with peripheral arterial disease reports that leg pain improves when dangling the legs over the bed. What does this indicate?
(A) Muscle strain
(B) Lymphedema
(C) Severe arterial insufficiency
(D) Improved venous return
Q534. A patient on warfarin therapy presents with spontaneous nosebleeds and INR of 5.8. What is the most appropriate action?
(A) Increase dose
(B) Continue therapy
(C) Encourage exercise
(D) Administer vitamin K
Q535. A patient with heart failure develops new confusion and low urine output. Blood pressure is 85/60 mmHg. What condition is suspected?
(A) Hyperthyroidism
(B) Dehydration only
(C) Cardiogenic shock
(D) Asthma exacerbation
Q536. A patient recovering from coronary artery bypass grafting develops sudden chest pressure and ST elevation. What is the priority?
(A) Encourage ambulation
(B) Prepare for urgent evaluation of graft patency
(C) Provide oral analgesics
(D) Schedule outpatient visit
Q537. A patient with chronic hypertension reports blurred vision and headache. Fundoscopic exam reveals retinal hemorrhages. What is the likely complication?
(A) Conjunctivitis
(B) Hypertensive retinopathy
(C) Glaucoma
(D) Cataract
Q538. A patient with infective endocarditis develops sudden abdominal pain and fever. What complication is most concerning?
(A) Constipation
(B) Splenic infarction
(C) Peptic ulcer
(D) Gastritis
Q539. A patient with dilated cardiomyopathy has an ejection fraction of 25%. What symptom is most expected?
(A) Increased exercise tolerance
(B) Weight loss only
(C) Polyuria
(D) Fatigue with minimal exertion

Q540. A patient with acute limb ischemia has pallor, pulselessness, and paralysis of the affected limb. What is the immediate priority?
(A) Elevate limb above heart
(B) Provide heat therapy
(C) Notify vascular surgeon urgently
(D) Apply compression bandage
Q541. A 59-year-old patient with a history of atrial fibrillation suddenly complains of severe left leg pain. The leg is pale, cold, and pulseless. What is the most likely cause?
(A) Deep vein thrombosis
(B) Cellulitis
(C) Chronic venous insufficiency
(D) Acute arterial embolism
Q542. A patient with chronic heart failure presents with increasing abdominal girth and right upper quadrant discomfort. What is the underlying mechanism?
(A) Renal calculi
(B) Gastric ulceration
(C) Hepatic congestion from right-sided failure
(D) Pulmonary congestion
Q543. A 72-year-old patient with severe coronary artery disease develops chest pain unrelieved by three doses of nitroglycerin. What is the priority action?
(A) Schedule clinic visit
(B) Take an antacid
(C) Activate emergency response system
(D) Advise rest at home
Q544. A patient receiving thrombolytic therapy for myocardial infarction suddenly develops hypotension and muffled heart sounds. What complication should be suspected?
(A) Pulmonary embolism
(B) Pericardial tamponade
(C) Dehydration
(D) Hypoglycemia
Q545. A patient with poorly controlled diabetes and hypertension reports chest discomfort during minimal exertion. What pathophysiologic process is most likely responsible?
(A) Pulmonary fibrosis
(B) Mitral valve prolapse
(C) Hyperthyroidism
(D) Coronary artery atherosclerosis
Q546. A patient admitted with infective endocarditis develops a new systolic murmur. What does this indicate?
(A) Electrolyte imbalance
(B) Improved cardiac function
(C) Valve damage progression
(D) Resolution of infection
Q547. A patient with heart failure is noncompliant with medications and presents with severe dyspnea and frothy sputum. What is the most likely immediate diagnosis?
(A) Acute pulmonary edema
(B) Pleural effusion
(C) Chronic bronchitis
(D) Pneumonia
Q548. A 67-year-old patient with long-standing hypertension presents with sudden severe headache and loss of consciousness. What is the most concerning diagnosis?
(A) Tension headache
(B) Hemorrhagic stroke
(C) Ischemic stroke
(D) Migraine
Q549. A patient with severe peripheral arterial disease has a nonhealing ulcer on the foot. What is the primary contributing factor?
(A) Hyperthyroidism
(B) Excessive hydration
(C) Reduced arterial perfusion
(D) Increased venous return
Q550. A patient with cardiomyopathy experiences palpitations and syncope. ECG reveals sustained ventricular tachycardia. What is the definitive long-term management strategy?
(A) Daily aspirin
(B) Implantable cardioverter-defibrillator
(C) Increase fluid intake
(D) Lifestyle modification only
Q551. A patient undergoing carotid artery stenting develops sudden facial droop and arm weakness during the procedure. What is the immediate priority?
(A) Assess neurologic status and notify team
(B) Reassure patient
(C) Administer oral fluids
(D) Continue procedure

Q552. A patient with chronic atrial fibrillation presents with rapid heart rate and hypotension. What is the most appropriate initial intervention?
(A) Immediate synchronized cardioversion
(B) Delay treatment
(C) Increase oral intake
(D) Encourage ambulation
Q553. A patient with untreated hyperlipidemia presents with stable angina. What structural change in coronary arteries is expected?
(A) Fibrous plaque formation
(B) Elastic dilation
(C) Smooth muscle relaxation
(D) Increased lumen diameter
Q554. A patient with advanced heart failure becomes increasingly lethargic and hypotensive. Urine output declines significantly. What complication is suspected?
(A) Hyperthyroidism
(B) Gastritis
(C) Asthma attack
(D) Cardiogenic shock
Q555. A patient with mitral stenosis reports worsening dyspnea and hemoptysis. What is the underlying cause?
(A) Increased systemic resistance
(B) Reduced pulmonary pressure
(C) Hypervolemia only
(D) Pulmonary venous congestion
Q556. A patient with uncontrolled hypertension is found to have left ventricular hypertrophy on echocardiogram. What is the primary risk associated with this condition?
(A) Progression to heart failure
(B) Decreased arrhythmia risk
(C) Improved cardiac efficiency
(D) Reduced myocardial oxygen demand
Q557. A patient with deep vein thrombosis on anticoagulation reports sudden severe abdominal pain. What complication should be considered?
(A) Internal bleeding
(B) Peptic ulcer
(C) Kidney stone
(D) Splenic infarction
Q558. A patient with chronic heart failure asks why daily weight monitoring is necessary. What is the best explanation?
(A) To assess bone density
(B) To detect early fluid retention
(C) To measure muscle growth
(D) To monitor blood glucose
Q559. A patient with severe coronary artery disease experiences chest pain at rest lasting 20 minutes. Troponin levels are elevated. What is the most likely diagnosis?
(A) Non-ST elevation myocardial infarction
(B) Gastroesophageal reflux
(C) Pericarditis
(D) Stable angina
Q560. A patient with peripheral arterial disease has diminished pulses and cool extremities. What lifestyle modification is most critical to slow disease progression?
(A) Prolonged bed rest
(B) High-fat diet
(C) Smoking cessation
(D) Increase sodium intake
Q561. A 63-year-old patient with a history of heart failure presents with sudden onset severe dyspnea and anxiety. Oxygen saturation is 82% on room air, and crackles are heard throughout the lung fields. What is the most appropriate initial intervention?
(A) Administer high-flow oxygen and position upright
(B) Lay the patient flat
(C) Encourage ambulation
(D) Provide oral fluids
Q562. A patient with long-standing atrial fibrillation stops taking anticoagulants and later presents with sudden vision loss in one eye. What is the most likely cause?
(A) Cataract formation
(B) Glaucoma
(C) Retinal artery embolism
(D) Macular degeneration
Q563. A patient undergoing dialysis reports chest pain and is found to have peaked T waves on ECG. What electrolyte imbalance is most likely responsible?
(A) Hyponatremia
(B) Hypokalemia

(C) Hypocalcemia
(D) Hyperkalemia

Q564. A patient with infective endocarditis complains of sudden left upper quadrant pain and fever. What complication should the nurse suspect?
(A) Appendicitis
(B) Splenic embolization
(C) Pancreatitis
(D) Gastritis

Q565. A patient with severe mitral stenosis becomes acutely short of breath during pregnancy. What physiologic change likely precipitated this episode?
(A) Decreased blood volume
(B) Lowered systemic resistance
(C) Increased cardiac output demand
(D) Reduced heart rate

Q566. A patient with a history of smoking and hypertension presents with sudden tearing chest pain and hypotension. Imaging confirms aortic dissection. What is the immediate management priority?
(A) Encourage walking
(B) Rapid blood pressure control
(C) Increase fluid intake
(D) Provide high-sodium diet

Q567. A patient with coronary artery disease develops chest pain while resting and has transient ST depression. Cardiac enzymes are normal. What condition is most consistent with these findings?
(A) Pericarditis
(B) Myocarditis
(C) Stable angina
(D) Unstable angina

Q568. A patient with chronic heart failure reports waking at night gasping for air. What term best describes this symptom?
(A) Claudication
(B) Orthostatic hypotension
(C) Paroxysmal nocturnal dyspnea
(D) Syncope

Q569. A patient receiving IV heparin therapy develops severe abdominal pain and hypotension. Hemoglobin levels drop significantly. What is the most likely cause?
(A) Gastroenteritis
(B) Kidney stone
(C) Internal bleeding
(D) Constipation

Q570. A patient with advanced peripheral arterial disease presents with blackened toes and foul odor. What is the most likely diagnosis?
(A) Wet gangrene
(B) Varicose veins
(C) Cellulitis
(D) Dry gangrene

Q571. A patient with severe cardiomyopathy is being evaluated for advanced therapy due to recurrent hospitalizations. What treatment option may be considered?
(A) Left ventricular assist device
(B) Discontinue medications
(C) Increased salt intake
(D) Bed rest only

Q572. A patient experiences sudden onset palpitations and dizziness. ECG reveals supraventricular tachycardia at 180 bpm. What is the initial nonpharmacologic intervention?
(A) Immediate defibrillation
(B) Provide oxygen only
(C) Administer diuretics
(D) Encourage coughing or Valsalva maneuver

Q573. A patient with chronic hypertension is diagnosed with left ventricular hypertrophy. What complication is this patient at highest risk for?
(A) Decreased arrhythmia risk
(B) Improved endurance
(C) Heart failure
(D) Hypotension

Q574. A patient with a prosthetic heart valve presents with fever and malaise. What complication should be suspected?
(A) Hyperlipidemia
(B) Dehydration
(C) Valve thrombosis
(D) Prosthetic valve endocarditis

Q575. A patient with uncontrolled diabetes reports calf pain when walking that resolves with rest. What is the most likely cause?
(A) Intermittent claudication
(B) Deep vein thrombosis
(C) Peripheral neuropathy

(D) Muscle strain

Q576. A patient collapses and is found pulseless with ventricular tachycardia on monitor. What is the immediate intervention?

(A) Oxygen by nasal cannula
(B) Defibrillation
(C) Oral beta-blocker
(D) Synchronized cardioversion

Q577. A patient with chronic heart failure is nonadherent to fluid restriction and presents with jugular venous distention and edema. What is the most likely result?

(A) Dehydration
(B) Hypernatremia only
(C) Hypovolemia
(D) Fluid overload

Q578. A patient with a history of myocardial infarction experiences new onset chest pain and has ST elevation in inferior leads. Which artery is most likely involved?

(A) Left anterior descending
(B) Right coronary artery
(C) Diagonal branch
(D) Left circumflex

Q579. A patient on long-term statin therapy reports muscle pain and weakness. What adverse effect should be suspected?

(A) Myopathy
(B) Arrhythmia
(C) Hyperglycemia
(D) Hypertension

Q580. A patient with severe heart failure is experiencing hypotension and cool extremities despite maximal medication therapy. What advanced treatment option may be considered?

(A) Bed rest only
(B) Discontinue monitoring
(C) Intra-aortic balloon pump
(D) Increase sodium intake

Q581. A 66-year-old patient with chronic atrial fibrillation presents with sudden severe abdominal pain out of proportion to physical findings. What complication should be suspected?

(A) Pancreatitis
(B) Acute gastritis
(C) Mesenteric arterial embolism
(D) Peptic ulcer disease

Q582. A patient with chronic heart failure reports increasing fatigue and confusion. Blood pressure is 78/50 mmHg and urine output is minimal. What condition is most likely developing?

(A) Septic shock
(B) Anaphylaxis
(C) Cardiogenic shock
(D) Hypovolemic shock

Q583. A patient with severe peripheral arterial disease reports constant foot pain that worsens at night and is relieved by dangling the leg. What does this indicate?

(A) Improved arterial flow
(B) Venous thrombosis
(C) Critical limb ischemia
(D) Muscle cramp

Q584. A patient receiving thrombolytic therapy for myocardial infarction develops sudden slurred speech and weakness. What is the immediate priority?

(A) Stop infusion and assess neurologic status
(B) Administer analgesics
(C) Continue infusion
(D) Encourage rest

Q585. A patient with dilated cardiomyopathy presents with worsening dyspnea and lower extremity edema despite medication adherence. Which mechanism explains symptom progression?

(A) Decreased systemic resistance
(B) Reduced preload
(C) Increased myocardial contractility
(D) Ventricular remodeling and dilation

Q586. A patient with a prosthetic mitral valve presents with fever and a new murmur. What is the most serious concern?

(A) Dehydration
(B) Prosthetic valve endocarditis
(C) Valve stenosis
(D) Hyperlipidemia

Q587. A patient with severe hypertension complains of chest pain and has ST depression on ECG. What is the likely underlying issue?

(A) Gastroesophageal reflux
(B) Myocardial ischemia due to increased demand

(C) Anxiety
(D) Pericarditis

Q588. A patient recovering from myocardial infarction suddenly develops a loud systolic murmur and pulmonary edema. What complication should be suspected?
(A) Pericardial effusion
(B) Hyperlipidemia
(C) Ventricular septal rupture
(D) Sinus tachycardia

Q589. A patient with long-standing diabetes presents with exertional chest discomfort that resolves with rest. What pathologic process is most likely present?
(A) Coronary artery atherosclerosis
(B) Pulmonary embolism
(C) Asthma
(D) Valve prolapse

Q590. A patient with chronic venous insufficiency presents with bilateral leg swelling and skin discoloration. What is the primary cause of these findings?
(A) Reduced cardiac output
(B) Hyperthyroidism
(C) Arterial occlusion
(D) Valve incompetence in veins

Q591. A patient with atrial fibrillation experiences rapid ventricular response and hypotension. What is the most urgent intervention?
(A) Delay treatment
(B) Provide analgesics
(C) Synchronized cardioversion
(D) Encourage hydration

Q592. A patient with severe heart failure develops worsening renal function. What is the most likely contributing factor?
(A) Reduced cardiac output
(B) Hyperthyroidism
(C) Improved perfusion
(D) Increased glomerular filtration

Q593. A patient with peripheral arterial disease develops sudden numbness and inability to move the foot. What does this signify?
(A) Advanced arterial occlusion
(B) Mild ischemia
(C) Muscle strain
(D) Venous congestion

Q594. A patient with hypertrophic cardiomyopathy reports syncope during exertion. What is the underlying cause?
(A) Hyperglycemia
(B) Reduced outflow from left ventricle
(C) Dehydration
(D) Increased venous return

Q595. A patient taking ACE inhibitors develops persistent dry cough. What is the most appropriate response?
(A) Assess severity and notify provider
(B) Increase dose
(C) Discontinue medication abruptly
(D) Ignore symptom

Q596. A patient with coronary artery disease presents with chest pain and elevated troponin but no ST elevation. What diagnosis is most consistent?
(A) Anxiety disorder
(B) Non-ST elevation myocardial infarction
(C) Pericarditis
(D) Stable angina

Q597. A patient with severe heart failure has cool extremities and delayed capillary refill. What does this indicate?
(A) Adequate perfusion
(B) Reduced systemic perfusion
(C) Hypervolemia
(D) Hypertension

Q598. A patient with untreated hyperlipidemia experiences sudden chest pain and is diagnosed with myocardial infarction. What was the primary underlying process?
(A) Plaque rupture and thrombosis
(B) Bronchospasm
(C) Valve calcification
(D) Dehydration

Q599. A patient with chronic atrial fibrillation asks about the purpose of beta-blocker therapy. What is the best explanation?
(A) Dissolve thrombus
(B) Control ventricular rate
(C) Prevent clot formation
(D) Increase cardiac output

Q600. A patient with advanced peripheral arterial disease presents with gangrene of the

toes and systemic signs of infection. What is the immediate priority?

(A) Urgent surgical evaluation
(B) Delay intervention
(C) Encourage ambulation
(D) Apply warm compresses

Answer Key and Explanation (501-600)

Q501. Answer: A

Explanation: Chronic hypertension creates sustained pressure overload against which the left ventricle must pump. This increases myocardial wall stress and stimulates compensatory thickening of the ventricular muscle. Over time, structural remodeling occurs to maintain cardiac output. Although initially adaptive, prolonged hypertrophy leads to decreased compliance and diastolic dysfunction. Eventually, this process may progress to heart failure.

Q502. Answer: D

Explanation: In atrial fibrillation, chaotic atrial activity prevents effective contraction. Blood pools in the atrial chambers, particularly the left atrial appendage. Stagnant blood promotes clot formation. These clots can dislodge and travel to cerebral arteries. Anticoagulation therapy significantly reduces this risk.

Q503. Answer: C

Explanation: During exertion, myocardial oxygen demand rises due to increased heart rate and contractility. If coronary arteries are narrowed, oxygen supply cannot meet demand. This mismatch leads to ischemia and chest discomfort. Rest reduces oxygen demand and relieves symptoms. Persistent imbalance may result in infarction.

Q504. Answer: B

Explanation: Systolic heart failure results from weakened ventricular contraction. Impaired contractility reduces stroke volume and cardiac output. Ventricular dilation often accompanies this dysfunction. Over time, neurohormonal activation worsens remodeling. Treatment focuses on improving contractile performance and reducing workload.

Q505. Answer: A

Explanation: ACE inhibitors block conversion of angiotensin I to angiotensin II. This reduces vasoconstriction and lowers systemic vascular resistance. Decreased afterload improves cardiac output in heart failure. These agents also limit adverse remodeling. Their use is associated with improved survival.

Q506. Answer: D

Explanation: Elevated LDL cholesterol penetrates damaged endothelium. Lipid accumulation triggers inflammatory responses within arterial walls. Foam cell formation and plaque development follow. Progressive narrowing impairs blood flow. Plaque rupture can lead to acute coronary syndromes.

Q507. Answer: B

Explanation: Left ventricular dysfunction causes blood to back up into the left atrium. This increases pulmonary venous and capillary pressures. Elevated hydrostatic pressure forces fluid into alveolar spaces. Gas exchange becomes impaired. Prompt treatment reduces congestion.

Q508. Answer: B

Explanation: Beta-blockers reduce heart rate and contractility. This lowers myocardial oxygen demand. Decreased workload limits infarct size and prevents arrhythmias. Long-term therapy improves survival. Careful titration is necessary to avoid bradycardia.

Q509. Answer: A

Explanation: Anticoagulants inhibit clotting cascade activity. They prevent further thrombus growth and reduce risk of embolization. Existing clots are gradually broken down by the body. Early initiation reduces complications. Monitoring ensures therapeutic effectiveness.

Q510. Answer: B

Explanation: Aortic stenosis restricts blood flow from the left ventricle. During exertion, systemic demand increases but cardiac output cannot rise adequately. Cerebral perfusion drops, leading to syncope. Left ventricular hypertrophy often develops. Valve replacement is definitive treatment.

Q511. Answer: B

Explanation: Right ventricular dysfunction causes blood to accumulate in systemic circulation. Elevated venous pressure pushes fluid into interstitial tissues. Peripheral edema and ascites may develop. Prolonged congestion affects organ function. Diuretics are often used for management.

Q512. Answer: A

Explanation: Sustained ischemia deprives myocardial tissue of oxygen. Within minutes, irreversible cellular damage begins. Early reperfusion salvages viable myocardium. Delays increase infarct size and mortality. Rapid intervention improves long-term outcomes.

Q513. Answer: B

Explanation: Electrolytes regulate cardiac action potentials. Imbalances disrupt depolarization and repolarization processes. Abnormal conduction predisposes to arrhythmias. Potassium disturbances are particularly significant. Correction restores electrical stability.

Q514. Answer: C

Explanation: Smoking introduces toxins that injure endothelial cells. Damaged endothelium promotes inflammation and plaque formation. Platelet activation and vasoconstriction also increase. Combined effects accelerate atherosclerosis. Smoking cessation significantly lowers risk.

Q515. Answer: A

Explanation: Diuretics increase renal excretion of sodium and water. This reduces circulating volume and venous pressure. Decreased preload alleviates pulmonary and systemic congestion. Symptom relief often occurs rapidly. Monitoring prevents electrolyte imbalance.

Q516. Answer: B

Explanation: Left bundle branch block alters normal depolarization pathways. This produces secondary ST-T changes on ECG. These changes can obscure signs of acute ischemia. Diagnosis of myocardial infarction becomes challenging. Clinical correlation is essential.

Q517. Answer: B

Explanation: Statins lower LDL and reduce inflammation within plaques. Stabilized plaques are less likely to rupture. This decreases risk of acute coronary events. Benefits extend beyond cholesterol reduction. Long-term therapy improves survival.

Q518. Answer: A

Explanation: Fluid accumulation in the pericardial sac exerts pressure on the heart. Ventricular filling during diastole becomes restricted. Reduced preload leads to decreased cardiac output. Hypotension and shock may develop. Emergent drainage is required.

Q519. Answer: A

Explanation: Cardiac rehabilitation combines supervised exercise, education, and counseling. It improves cardiovascular fitness and quality of life. Structured programs reduce recurrence risk. Gradual progression ensures safety. Multidisciplinary support enhances outcomes.

Q520. Answer: C

Explanation: Insulin resistance leads to metabolic abnormalities. Elevated glucose and lipids damage endothelial cells. Inflammatory processes accelerate plaque formation. Associated hypertension and dyslipidemia further increase risk. Comprehensive management reduces cardiovascular events.

Q521. Answer: A

Explanation: Prolonged crushing chest pain with radiation suggests acute myocardial infarction. Early ECG acquisition is critical to identify ischemic changes. Rapid diagnosis allows timely reperfusion therapy. Delayed evaluation increases myocardial damage. Immediate cardiac monitoring improves patient outcomes.

Q522. Answer: D

Explanation: Rapid weight gain and crackles indicate fluid overload. Excess sodium intake may contribute to worsening congestion. Reinforcing dietary compliance helps prevent further retention. Early intervention may avoid hospitalization. Monitoring daily weight trends is essential in management.

Q523. Answer: C

Explanation: Pink frothy sputum suggests acute pulmonary edema. Hypoxia requires immediate oxygen therapy. Improving oxygenation stabilizes vital organs. Positioning upright also assists breathing. Rapid diuretic administration may follow stabilization.

Q524. Answer: C

Explanation: Atrial fibrillation predisposes to thrombus formation in the atria. Without anticoagulation, emboli can travel to cerebral arteries. Sudden neurologic deficits are characteristic of ischemic stroke. Immediate activation of stroke protocol is required. Early intervention reduces disability.

Q525. Answer: C

Explanation: Severe back pain and hypotension after catheterization suggest internal bleeding. Retroperitoneal hemorrhage is a known complication of femoral access. Rapid recognition prevents shock progression. Vital signs and hemoglobin levels require monitoring. Immediate provider notification is critical.

Q526. Answer: C

Explanation: Hypertensive emergency requires careful blood pressure reduction. Rapid lowering may compromise cerebral perfusion. Controlled reduction prevents further end-organ damage. Intravenous medications are titrated closely. Continuous monitoring is essential.

Q527. Answer: C

Explanation: Sudden chest pain and rapid breathing in a patient with DVT suggest embolization. A clot may have traveled to the pulmonary arteries. This impairs gas exchange and can be life-threatening. Prompt diagnostic evaluation is necessary. Early anticoagulation improves prognosis.

Q528. Answer: A

Explanation: Aortic stenosis limits forward blood flow during exertion. Cardiac output cannot meet systemic demands. Reduced cerebral perfusion leads to syncope. This is a classic symptom of advanced disease. Valve intervention may be required.

Q529. Answer: D

Explanation: Tearing chest pain radiating to the back is characteristic of aortic dissection. Blood pressure discrepancy suggests involvement of major vessels. Immediate imaging is required. Rapid intervention can be life-saving. Delays increase mortality risk.

Q530. Answer: A

Explanation: Elevated potassium indicates hyperkalemia. Spironolactone can cause potassium retention. Severe hyperkalemia increases arrhythmia risk. Immediate provider notification is necessary. Cardiac monitoring should be initiated.

Q531. Answer: A

Explanation: Mitral regurgitation allows blood to flow backward during systole. Increased volume in the left atrium causes enlargement. Over time, pulmonary congestion may develop. Symptoms reflect decreased forward output. Surgical correction may be necessary.

Q532. Answer: B

Explanation: Ventricular fibrillation is a life-threatening arrhythmia. Immediate defibrillation restores organized rhythm. Delayed shock decreases survival rates. CPR should continue until shock is delivered. Rapid response improves outcomes.

Q533. Answer: C

Explanation: Dangling legs increases arterial perfusion by gravity. Relief of rest pain suggests advanced arterial disease. This is often seen in critical limb ischemia. Immediate vascular evaluation is required. Tissue viability may be compromised.

Q534. Answer: D

Explanation: Elevated INR increases bleeding risk. Nosebleeds indicate active hemorrhagic tendency. Vitamin K reverses excessive anticoagulation. Monitoring ensures stabilization. Dose adjustment will likely be necessary.

Q535. Answer: C

Explanation: Hypotension with reduced urine output indicates poor perfusion. Confusion suggests cerebral hypoxia. Cardiogenic shock results from severe pump failure. Immediate hemodynamic support is needed. Early intervention reduces mortality.

Q536. Answer: B

Explanation: New ST elevation after bypass surgery suggests graft occlusion. Rapid evaluation prevents further myocardial damage. Immediate cardiology consultation is necessary. Time-sensitive intervention improves outcomes. Delays increase infarct size.

Q537. Answer: B

Explanation: Persistent high blood pressure damages retinal vessels. Hemorrhages and exudates indicate advanced disease. Vision disturbances may occur. Strict blood pressure control prevents progression. Regular monitoring is essential.

Q538. Answer: B

Explanation: Septic emboli from infected valves may lodge in abdominal organs. Splenic infarction causes acute pain and fever. Early detection guides management. Continued antibiotic therapy is essential. Complications require prompt evaluation.

Q539. Answer: D

Explanation: Reduced ejection fraction indicates severe systolic dysfunction. Cardiac output is insufficient to meet demands. Patients experience fatigue and dyspnea. Activity tolerance decreases significantly. Guideline-directed therapy improves symptoms.

Q540. Answer: C

Explanation: The presence of pallor, pulselessness, and paralysis indicates severe ischemia. Tissue necrosis may occur quickly. Urgent surgical intervention is required. Delays can result in permanent limb loss. Rapid restoration of perfusion is critical.

Q541. Answer: D

Explanation: Atrial fibrillation predisposes to clot formation in the atria. An embolus can travel through systemic circulation and lodge in a peripheral artery. Sudden onset pain with pallor and absent pulse indicates acute arterial occlusion. This is a vascular emergency requiring immediate intervention. Rapid restoration of blood flow is essential to prevent tissue necrosis.

Q542. Answer: C

Explanation: Right-sided heart failure leads to systemic venous congestion. Blood backs up into the hepatic circulation, causing liver enlargement and discomfort. Ascites may also develop due to elevated venous pressures. These findings reflect worsening right ventricular dysfunction. Diuretic therapy and fluid management are typically required.

Q543. Answer: C

Explanation: Chest pain unrelieved by nitroglycerin suggests possible myocardial infarction. Immediate emergency activation ensures rapid medical evaluation. Time-sensitive reperfusion therapy may be necessary. Delays increase myocardial injury. Prompt intervention improves survival.

Q544. Answer: B

Explanation: Hypotension with muffled heart sounds suggests fluid accumulation in the pericardial sac. Thrombolytic therapy can increase bleeding risk, including into the pericardium. Tamponade impairs ventricular filling and reduces cardiac output. Rapid diagnosis and pericardiocentesis are critical. Early recognition prevents cardiovascular collapse.

Q545. Answer: D

Explanation: Diabetes and hypertension accelerate atherosclerotic plaque formation. Narrowed coronary arteries limit oxygen supply during exertion. Even minimal activity can precipitate ischemia. This pattern suggests progressive coronary disease. Aggressive risk factor management is essential.

Q546. Answer: C

Explanation: Infective endocarditis can destroy valve leaflets. A new murmur suggests worsening regurgitation. Structural damage may impair cardiac output. Echocardiography is required to evaluate severity. Early treatment prevents further complications.

Q547. Answer: A

Explanation: Noncompliance can precipitate acute decompensation. Frothy sputum and severe dyspnea are classic for pulmonary edema. Fluid accumulates in alveoli due to elevated pressures. Immediate oxygen and diuretics are required. Early management reduces respiratory failure risk.

Q548. Answer: B

Explanation: Severe headache with sudden collapse suggests intracranial hemorrhage. Chronic hypertension weakens cerebral vessels. Rupture leads to bleeding within brain tissue. Immediate neuroimaging is essential. Rapid intervention may limit damage.

Q549. Answer: C

Explanation: Arterial insufficiency limits oxygen delivery to tissues. Poor perfusion delays wound healing. Chronic ischemia may lead to ulcer formation. Vascular assessment guides treatment options. Revascularization may be necessary.

Q550. Answer: B

Explanation: Sustained ventricular tachycardia in structural heart disease carries high sudden death risk. An implantable cardioverter-defibrillator detects and terminates life-threatening arrhythmias. This significantly reduces mortality. Pharmacologic therapy may complement device use. Careful follow-up is required.

Q551. Answer: A

Explanation: Sudden neurologic changes during carotid intervention suggest embolization. Immediate assessment determines stroke severity. Rapid response may allow early treatment. Delays increase risk of permanent deficits. Continuous monitoring is essential.

Q552. Answer: A

Explanation: Hemodynamic instability in atrial fibrillation requires urgent rhythm control. Synchronized cardioversion restores organized electrical activity. Prompt intervention stabilizes blood pressure. Continuous monitoring is necessary. Early treatment prevents deterioration.

Q553. Answer: A

Explanation: Elevated lipids contribute to plaque buildup in arterial walls. Fibrous caps develop over lipid cores. Progressive narrowing restricts blood flow. Stable angina reflects fixed obstruction. Risk modification slows progression.

Q554. Answer: D

Explanation: Reduced perfusion from pump failure leads to hypotension and oliguria. Lethargy indicates decreased cerebral perfusion. Cardiogenic shock is a life-threatening emergency. Hemodynamic support is required. Early aggressive management improves survival.

Q555. Answer: D

Explanation: Mitral stenosis obstructs blood flow from left atrium to ventricle. Pressure increases in pulmonary circulation. Capillary rupture may cause hemoptysis. Chronic congestion leads to progressive dyspnea. Intervention may include valve repair or replacement.

Q556. Answer: A

Explanation: Persistent pressure overload causes myocardial thickening. Over time, compliance decreases and diastolic dysfunction develops. Eventually systolic impairment may occur. This progression increases risk of heart failure. Effective blood pressure control can prevent worsening.

Q557. Answer: A

Explanation: Anticoagulation increases bleeding risk. Sudden abdominal pain may indicate internal hemorrhage. Monitoring hemoglobin and vital signs is essential. Rapid evaluation prevents shock. Dose adjustment may be required.

Q558. Answer: B

Explanation: Small increases in weight often reflect fluid accumulation. Early detection allows prompt adjustment of therapy. This helps prevent acute decompensation. Daily monitoring provides consistent trends. Patient involvement improves self-management.

Q559. Answer: A

Explanation: Elevated troponin indicates myocardial injury. Chest pain at rest suggests acute coronary syndrome. Absence of ST elevation differentiates this from STEMI. Prompt antiplatelet and anticoagulant therapy is required. Early intervention reduces complications.

Q560. Answer: C

Explanation: Smoking accelerates atherosclerosis and vasoconstriction. Continued use worsens arterial narrowing. Cessation improves endothelial function and circulation. It significantly reduces cardiovascular events. Behavioral support enhances success rates.

Q561. Answer: A

Explanation: Severe dyspnea with diffuse crackles suggests acute pulmonary edema. Hypoxia must be corrected immediately to prevent organ damage. Upright positioning reduces venous return and pulmonary congestion. Supplemental oxygen improves gas exchange. Rapid stabilization is essential before further interventions.

Q562. Answer: C

Explanation: Atrial fibrillation increases risk of thrombus formation. An embolus can travel to the retinal artery, causing sudden vision loss. This is a medical emergency. Immediate evaluation is required to attempt vision preservation. Consistent anticoagulation reduces such risks.

Q563. Answer: D

Explanation: Dialysis patients are prone to potassium fluctuations. Peaked T waves are a classic sign of elevated potassium levels. Hyperkalemia can progress to life-threatening arrhythmias. Immediate treatment is required to stabilize cardiac membranes. Continuous cardiac monitoring is essential.

Q564. Answer: B

Explanation: Vegetations from infected heart valves may embolize systemically. The spleen is a common target for septic emboli. Sudden abdominal pain and fever suggest infarction. Imaging confirms diagnosis. Ongoing antibiotic therapy is critical.

Q565. Answer: C

Explanation: Pregnancy increases blood volume and cardiac output demands. Mitral stenosis limits flow from left atrium to ventricle. Elevated atrial pressure worsens pulmonary congestion. Acute dyspnea may occur. Close monitoring is required during pregnancy.

Q566. Answer: B

Explanation: Aortic dissection requires prompt reduction of shear stress on the vessel wall. Controlling blood pressure prevents extension of the tear. Intravenous antihypertensives are typically used. Continuous monitoring is necessary. Early surgical consultation is essential.

Q567. Answer: D

Explanation: Chest pain at rest with transient ECG changes suggests unstable angina. Normal enzymes indicate no myocardial necrosis yet. This condition is part of acute coronary syndrome. Urgent evaluation and medical therapy are required. Early intervention reduces progression to infarction.

Q568. Answer: C

Explanation: Sudden nighttime breathlessness is characteristic of paroxysmal nocturnal dyspnea. Fluid redistribution increases pulmonary congestion during sleep. Patients often sit upright for relief. This indicates worsening left ventricular dysfunction. Treatment adjustment may be necessary.

Q569. Answer: C

Explanation: Heparin increases bleeding risk by inhibiting clot formation. Sudden abdominal pain with hypotension suggests hemorrhage. A falling hemoglobin level confirms blood loss. Immediate discontinuation and reversal may be necessary. Rapid assessment prevents shock.

Q570. Answer: A

Explanation: Blackened tissue with foul odor indicates infection and tissue necrosis. Wet gangrene involves bacterial invasion and requires urgent care. Delayed treatment may lead to systemic infection. Surgical evaluation is required. Early intervention reduces mortality.

Q571. Answer: A

Explanation: Advanced heart failure may require mechanical circulatory support. A left ventricular assist device improves cardiac output. It can serve as bridge to transplant or destination therapy. Careful patient selection is required. This option improves survival and quality of life.

Q572. Answer: D

Explanation: Vagal maneuvers can terminate certain supraventricular tachycardias. These techniques increase parasympathetic tone. They may restore normal rhythm without medication. If ineffective, pharmacologic therapy follows. Continuous monitoring is necessary.

Q573. Answer: C

Explanation: Left ventricular hypertrophy initially compensates for pressure overload. Over time, stiffened myocardium impairs filling. This leads to diastolic dysfunction and heart failure. Arrhythmias may also develop. Blood pressure control prevents progression.

Q574. Answer: D

Explanation: Prosthetic valves increase infection risk. Fever and malaise may indicate endocarditis. Early blood cultures are necessary. Prompt antibiotic therapy prevents valve destruction. Delayed treatment increases mortality.

Q575. Answer: A

Explanation: Diabetes accelerates atherosclerosis in peripheral arteries. Reduced blood flow during exertion causes ischemic pain. Rest decreases oxygen demand and relieves symptoms. This pattern defines intermittent claudication. Lifestyle and medical management are essential.

Q576. Answer: B

Explanation: Pulseless ventricular tachycardia is treated as cardiac arrest. Immediate defibrillation is required. High-quality CPR should continue until shock is delivered. Delays reduce survival rates. Early intervention improves outcomes.

Q577. Answer: D

Explanation: Excess fluid intake increases circulating volume. In heart failure, the heart cannot manage additional preload effectively. Venous congestion develops, leading to edema and JVD. Adherence to fluid restriction is critical. Education reinforces self-management.

Q578. Answer: B

Explanation: Inferior leads correspond to the inferior wall of the heart. This region is commonly supplied by the right coronary artery. ST elevation indicates acute injury. Rapid reperfusion therapy is necessary. Early treatment limits infarct size.

Q579. Answer: A

Explanation: Statins can cause muscle-related side effects. Myopathy presents with pain and weakness. Severe cases may progress to rhabdomyolysis. Laboratory evaluation of muscle enzymes may be necessary. Dose adjustment or discontinuation may be required.

Q580. Answer: C

Explanation: Intra-aortic balloon pump supports circulation by improving coronary perfusion and reducing afterload. It is used in severe cases of cardiogenic shock. Mechanical support stabilizes hemodynamics temporarily. It serves as bridge to further intervention. Careful monitoring is essential.

Q581. Answer: C

Explanation: Atrial fibrillation predisposes to thrombus formation that can embolize to systemic arteries. Sudden severe abdominal pain disproportionate to examination findings suggests mesenteric ischemia. This condition compromises intestinal blood flow. Rapid diagnosis is essential to prevent bowel necrosis. Immediate vascular evaluation is required.

Q582. Answer: C

Explanation: Severe hypotension with reduced urine output indicates inadequate organ perfusion. In the setting of heart failure, pump failure is the likely cause. Cardiogenic shock results from markedly decreased cardiac output. Confusion reflects cerebral hypoperfusion. Immediate hemodynamic support is required.

Q583. Answer: C

Explanation: Rest pain indicates severely compromised arterial perfusion. Relief by dependency suggests gravity-assisted blood flow. This is characteristic of critical limb ischemia. Tissue viability is at risk. Urgent vascular intervention may be necessary.

Q584. Answer: A

Explanation: Sudden neurologic changes during thrombolytic therapy suggest intracranial hemorrhage. Immediate discontinuation reduces further bleeding risk. Rapid neurologic assessment is critical. Early imaging confirms diagnosis. Prompt action can be life-saving.

Q585. Answer: D

Explanation: Dilated cardiomyopathy involves progressive ventricular enlargement. Remodeling reduces systolic function over time. Decreased ejection fraction leads to congestion. Symptoms worsen despite therapy. Advanced management strategies may be required.

Q586. Answer: B

Explanation: Fever and new murmur in a patient with prosthetic valve raise suspicion for infection. Endocarditis can damage valve structure and impair function. Blood cultures are necessary for diagnosis. Early antibiotic therapy is critical. Delayed treatment increases mortality risk.

Q587. Answer: B

Explanation: Severe hypertension increases myocardial oxygen demand. ST depression suggests subendocardial ischemia. The heart struggles to meet oxygen requirements. Early treatment reduces risk of infarction. Blood pressure control is essential.

Q588. Answer: C

Explanation: Mechanical complications can occur after infarction. Septal rupture causes abnormal left-to-right shunting. This leads to acute heart failure and pulmonary congestion. Rapid diagnosis is critical. Surgical intervention is often required.

Q589. Answer: A

Explanation: Diabetes accelerates plaque formation in coronary arteries. Reduced blood flow during exertion causes ischemia. Rest decreases oxygen demand and relieves pain. This pattern is typical of stable angina. Risk factor management is essential.

Q590. Answer: D

Explanation: Venous valve dysfunction leads to blood pooling in lower extremities. Increased venous pressure causes edema and skin changes. Chronic inflammation may result in hyperpigmentation. Elevation and compression therapy are common treatments. Early management prevents ulcer formation.

Q591. Answer: C

Explanation: Hemodynamic instability in atrial fibrillation requires immediate rhythm correction. Synchronized cardioversion restores coordinated contraction. This improves cardiac output and blood pressure. Rapid intervention prevents organ hypoperfusion. Continuous monitoring is required.

Q592. Answer: A

Explanation: Decreased cardiac output reduces renal blood flow. Poor perfusion impairs kidney function. This condition is often referred to as cardiorenal syndrome. Monitoring renal parameters is important. Treatment focuses on optimizing circulation.

Q593. Answer: A

Explanation: Neurologic deficits indicate severe ischemia. Motor and sensory loss reflect inadequate perfusion. Tissue necrosis may occur quickly. Immediate surgical evaluation is necessary. Rapid restoration of blood flow is critical.

Q594. Answer: B

Explanation: Hypertrophic cardiomyopathy causes obstruction of left ventricular outflow. During exertion, obstruction worsens. Cerebral perfusion decreases, leading to syncope. Sudden cardiac death risk is elevated. Close monitoring is required.

Q595. Answer: A

Explanation: Dry cough is a known side effect of ACE inhibitors. It results from bradykinin accumulation. Assessing severity helps determine need for medication change. Alternative agents may be considered. Communication with provider ensures safe management.

Q596. Answer: B

Explanation: Elevated troponin indicates myocardial injury. Absence of ST elevation differentiates this from STEMI. This represents an acute coronary syndrome. Prompt medical therapy reduces infarct expansion. Monitoring is required to prevent complications.

Q597. Answer: B

Explanation: Cool extremities reflect vasoconstriction and poor blood flow. Delayed capillary refill indicates decreased perfusion. These findings are common in low-output states. Immediate assessment is necessary. Treatment aims to improve circulation.

Q598. Answer: A

Explanation: Hyperlipidemia promotes plaque formation in coronary arteries. Plaque rupture exposes thrombogenic material. Thrombus formation occludes blood flow. Myocardial tissue becomes ischemic and necrotic. Early reperfusion limits damage.

Q599. Answer: B

Explanation: Beta-blockers slow atrioventricular conduction. This controls ventricular response in atrial fibrillation. Rate control improves symptoms and hemodynamics. Anticoagulants are used for stroke prevention. Combined therapy improves outcomes.

Q600. Answer: A

Explanation: Gangrene with systemic infection indicates severe tissue necrosis. Sepsis risk is high. Immediate surgical consultation is necessary. Debridement or amputation may be required. Early intervention prevents life-threatening complications.

Made in United States
Orlando, FL
04 November 2026

90206047R00083